# THE SANCTITY-OF-LIFE DOCTRINE
## IN MEDICINE

THE

# Sanctity-of-Life
# Doctrine in Medicine

A CRITIQUE

HELGA KUHSE

CLARENDON PRESS · OXFORD
1987

Oxford University Press, Walton Street, Oxford OX2 6DP

Oxford New York Toronto Melbourne Auckland
Delhi Bombay Calcutta Madras Karachi
Petaling Jaya Singapore Hong Kong Tokyo
Nairobi Dar es Salaam Cape Town

Associated companies in Beirut Berlin Ibadan Nicosia

OXFORD is a trade mark of Oxford University Press

Published in the United States
by Oxford University Press, New York

British Library Cataloguing in Publication Data
Kuhse, Helga
The sanctity-of-life doctrine in medicine:
a critique.
1. Euthanasia—Moral and ethical aspects
I. Title
174'.24      R726
ISBN 0-19-824943-8

Library of Congress Cataloging in Publication Data
Kuhse, Helga.
The sanctity-of-life doctrine in medicine.
Bibliography: p.
Includes index.
1. Medical ethics. 2. Life and death, Power over.
3. Quality of life. I. Title. [DNLM: 1. Ethics,
Medical. 2. Euthanasia. 3. Quality of life.
W 50 K96s]
R724.K83   1987      174'.24      87-7904
ISBN 0-19-824943-8

Printed in Great Britain
at the University Printing House, Oxford
by David Stanford
Printer to the University

FOR BILL

# PREFACE

FEW moral convictions are more deeply ingrained than that of the sanctity of human life. In medicine, 'sanctity of life' has traditionally stood for the absolute inviolability of human life and its equal value. But unprecedented advances in medical science and technology raise some old and troubling questions with renewed urgency: must all human lives, irrespective of their quality or kind, always be prolonged, or are there times when it is permissible to let—or help—a patient die?

In the past, answers to these questions have often been phrased in terms of a qualified sanctity-of-life view: that it is always wrong intentionally to terminate a patient's life, but that it is sometimes permissible for a doctor to let a patient die.

This book is a philosophical critique of the sanctity-of-life view. I argue that the principles espoused by those who subscribe to the sanctity-of-life view are philosophically flawed and lead to indefensible practical consequences—such as the making of life and death decisions on morally irrelevant grounds.

The arguments by which I reach these conclusions are sometimes complex; the detailed List of Contents provides a guide and a summary. The first four chapters of the book are negative: they constitute a critique which should lead us to reject the view that has influenced our thoughts and practices for too long. Chapter 5 is a brief positive contribution to the debate. It provides a sketch of a quality-of-life ethic offered in the belief that philosophers should not only interpret and criticize the world, but point the way towards change.

# ACKNOWLEDGEMENTS

THIS book owes much to my friend and colleague Peter Singer. He was the source of valuable encouragement, of constructive criticisms, and of many helpful suggestions. At the same time, I should like to acknowledge an older debt and thank him for having stimulated my interest in ethics when I was fortunate to have him as my teacher during my undergraduate and postgraduate years at Monash University. Without him, this book might never have been written.

I am also deeply indebted to a number of other people for helpful comments and criticisms: Professor Joseph Fletcher and Professor R. M. Hare, who were the examiners of what was then my Ph.D. thesis; Dr Jefferson McMahan, who acted as one of the readers for Oxford University Press, and Dr Robert Young who scrutinized very carefully a final draft of the book. This book is much better as a result of their perceptive and valuable criticisms and suggestions.

HELGA KUHSE

# CORRIGENDA

p. 92    line 25, add footnote:

[16a] See also Suzanne Uniack's discussion of Glover's interpretation of this case ('The Doctrine of Double Effect', *The Thomist* 48:2 (April 1984), 196–7). Uniacke points out that Jonathan Glover is wrong when he assumes (in *Causing Death and Saving Lives*) that the shooting of the trapped man 'would have been condemned by the double effect doctrine'. Rather, Uniacke suggests, this and similar actions 'are not condemned by the Doctrine of Double Effect. They are condemned by the Catholic teaching that it is never permissible intentionally to take innocent human life . . .'.

p. 93    line 4, after 'sanctity-of-life doctrine', add:

Here I should like to acknowledge a debt to Suzanne Uniacke, whose careful analysis of The PDE has been most valuable in shaping my thoughts on the doctrine. From time to time, I shall make reference to Ms. Uniacke's work.[16b]

p. 93    foot of page, add footnote:

[16b] Uniacke: 'The Doctrine of Double Effect', 188–218.

p. 96    line 16, after 'importance', add footnote:

[21a] In my analysis of condition 2 of the PDE on this and the next page, I am indebted to Uniacke: 'The Doctrine of Double Effect', 206–9.

p. 100    line 12, this sentence should begin:

As Uniacke points out,[32a] to exclude such sophistical . . .

p. 100    foot of page, add footnote:

[32a] Uniacke: 'The Doctrine of Double Effect', 208–9.

p. 131    line 7, after 'lethal injection', add footnote:

[97a] Uniacke:'The Doctrine of Double Effect', 208, makes this point.

p. 150 line 27, after 'action', add footnote:

[131a] Uniacke:'The Doctrine of Double Effect', 212–15.

p. 154    line 31, after 'blameworthiness', add footnote:

[138a] On the necessity to distinguish between responsibility and blameworthiness, and the criticism of some recent accounts of responsibility on this basis, see Uniacke:'The Doctrine of Double Effect', 216.

## Corrigenda

p. 155    line 15, after 'good actions', add footnote:

[138b] Uniacke:'The Doctrine of Double Effect', 212.

p. 155    line 36, after *'permissibility'* of an action', add footnote:

[139a] On Anscombe's mistaken understanding of double effect and her confusion of responsibility and blameworthiness see Uniacke:'The Doctrine of Double Effect', 213-15.

p. 235    Index, *for* Uniacke, S. M. 156 *read:*

# CONTENTS

# I

# The 'Sanctity-of-Life Doctrine'
# and Ethical Consistency

To persons who are not murderers, concentration camp adminis-
trators, or dreamers of sadistic fantasies, the inviolability of human life
seems to be so self-evident that it might appear pointless to inquire into
it. To inquire into it is embarrassing as well because, once raised, the
question seems to commit us to beliefs we do not wish to espouse and
to confront us with contradictions which seem to deny what is self-
evident.

> Edward Shils: 'The Sanctity of Life', in D. H. Labby: *Life or
> Death: Ethics and Options*, 1968

... and if I say again that daily to discourse about virtue, and of those
other things about which you hear me examining myself and others, is
the greatest good of man, and that the unexamined life is no life for a
human being, you are still less likely to believe me.

> Socrates in Plato's *Apology*

## I.I  INTRODUCTION: THE 'SANCTITY OF LIFE'

'THE unexamined life is not worth living.' With these words,
Socrates—contemporary of Hippocrates and the first great moral
philosopher of western civilization—stated the creed of reflective
men and women, and set the task for ethics: to seek, with the help of
reason, a consistent and defensible approach to life and its moral
dilemmas.

Ethical inquiry is important to us when we are unsure of the
direction in which we are heading. Like philosophy, it thrives on self-
doubt. Athens after the death of Pericles and England after the death
of Charles I are good examples. So is our time.

'New philosophy calls all in doubt' wrote John Donne in the wake
of the Copernican Revolution and a few decades before Charles I's
violent death, suggesting that new thoughts had challenged old

2 *The Sanctity of Life and Ethical Consistency*

practices.[1] Today, new practices in the biomedical sciences are challenging old thoughts: 'New medicine calls all in doubt.'

Few moral convictions are more deeply ingrained than that of the sanctity of life. However, if plausible once, the view that life is a divine gift (bestowed, sustained, and finally reclaimed by God) is now more difficult to maintain. Sophisticated modern medical science and technology has given us the means to achieve a continuously increasing control over our lives. Not only can doctors and scientists now initiate individual human life by means of *in vitro* fertilization and embryo transfer, but death can, quite often, be kept waiting by the bed or machine. This means that even if we are ultimately unable to conquer death, we have a lot to say about the conditions and time of its occurrence.

With this an old question is raised with renewed urgency: must human life, regardless of its quality of kind, always be preserved? Is it the physician's duty to sustain indefinitely the life of an irreversibly brain-damaged person by way of artificial respiration and intravenous feeding? Must the physician engage in 'heroic' efforts, that is, employ all of modern medicine's devices to add another few weeks, days, or even hours to the life of a terminally ill and suffering cancer patient? Must active treatment be instigated with regard to babies born so defective that their future promises little more than continuous suffering or mere vegetative existence? Or is it sometimes permissible to let a patient die?

These questions are not new, but they are today posed with relentless clarity and urgency. Given that we *can* sustain lives such as the above, *ought* such lives to be sustained—and if not, why not? And if not all lives need or ought to be sustained, would it then be permissible to shorten them by direct means?

Traditionally, answers to these questions have been phrased in terms of what I want to call the 'qualified sanctity-of-life doctrine': the view that it is always wrong to kill a patient, but that it is sometimes permissible to let a patient die.

Here we should note that I shall not, when speaking of the sanctity-of-life doctrine, be using the term 'sanctity' in a specifically religious sense. While the doctrine may well have its source in theology (as I shall suggest in Section 1.4), I am not concerned with the question of whether or not the doctrine is true to some theological tradition or other, but rather with the question of whether it can be defended on

[1] John Donne: 'The First Anniversary', reprinted in various anthologies.

non-theological grounds. The sanctity-of-life doctrine has become part of conventional secular morality, and it is as such that it is most influential today.

The sanctity-of-life doctrine needs to be distinguished from other views appealing to some principle or principles of the sanctity of life or the wrongness of killing. Albert Schweitzer,[2] some environmentalists, Buddhist, and Jains advocate an ethics of reverence for all life. Many of us think that it is wrong wantonly to kill at least some non-human animals, and most of us believe that human life has some very special value and that it is wrong (at least prima facie) to kill other people. To the extent that we hold such beliefs, we share in a doctrine, or rather a group of doctrines, that are central in discussions involving the sanctity of life and the wrongness of killing. However, even if the various ideas that life has sanctity (or demands respect) are often impossibly vague and misleading, the sanctity-of-life doctrine as it underlies the practice of medicine and as it is enshrined by the law can be given a definite outline.[3]

Medicine does not concern itself with life in all its forms, nor with the wrongness of killing as such: it leaves this to the biologist or the philosopher. Doctors have not generally campaigned for a new environmental ethic nor argued for vegetarianism, and non-human life is sacrificed in experiments directed at prolonging and improving human life. In medicine, 'Sanctity of life' means the sanctity of *human* life—that is, the bodily life possessed by us between conception or birth and death.[4]

Traditional medicine, entwined with religion since the time of Hippocrates, does not, for example, draw philosophical distinctions between different kinds or types of life, such as the life of a human organism and the life of a 'person' (in the sense of a conscious or self-conscious being). Along with many other philosophers, I regard these

[2] Albert Schweitzer: *Civilization and Ethics*, 3rd edn. (London: Black, 1949).

[3] The extreme vagueness of the sanctity-of-life doctrine has repeatedly been pointed out; see, for example, Marvin Kohl: 'The Sanctity-of-Life Principle', in Marvin Kohl (ed.): *The Morality of Killing: Sanctity-of-Life, Abortion and Euthanasia* (London: Peter Owen, 1974), 3–23; William K. Frankena: 'The Ethics of Respect for Life', in Stephen F. Barker (ed.): *Respect for Life in Medicine, Philosophy, and the Law* (Baltimore: Johns Hopkins University Press, 1977), 24–62; Edward W. Keyserlingk: *Sanctity of Life or Quality of Life in the Context of Ethics, Medicine and Law*). Study written for the Law Reform Commission of Canada. (Ottawa: Law Reform Commission 1979, 9–47.)

[4] See Owsei Temkin: 'Respect for Life in the History of Medicine', in Stephen F. Barker (ed.): *Respect for Life in Medicine*, 15–16.

distinctions—which I shall be discussing in greater detail in Chapter 5—as necessary if questions as to the foundation of a right to life or the wrongness of killing are to be answered in a non-arbitrary way. For medical professionals and their legal colleagues, all human life is in theory—although, as we shall see, not always in practice—equally valuable and inviolable. Amongst other things, doctors have thus pledged to 'maintain the utmost respect for human life from the time of conception',[5] and a typical code of ethics for nurses states: 'The nurses' respect for the worth and dignity of the individual human being extends throughout the entire life cycle, from birth to death.'[6]

If 'life' in medicine thus means 'bodily human life', 'sanctity of' or 'respect for' life means that all bodily human life, irrespective of its quality or kind, is equally valuable and inviolable. This means that life and death decisions must not, on this view, be based on quality-of-life considerations.

Those who subscribe to the sanctity-of-life view do not, however, generally hold that every patient's life that can be prolonged ought to be prolonged by all available medical means. Rather, what supporters of the sanctity-of-life doctrine typically suggest is that there are times when an agent may legitimately allow a patient to die. In other words, they subscribe to what I called above the *qualified* sanctity-of-life view, which I shall outline in Section 1.5. This raises two important questions regarding the fundamental tenets of the sanctity-of-life view—that all human life is inviolable and equally valuable.

—Can a limited duty of life-preservation consistently be combined with the view that all human life is inviolable and that the intentional termination of human life is always wrong?
—Are those who posit a limited duty of life-preservation consistent in according an equal value to all human lives, or are they making implicit quality-of-life judgements when they suggest that not all lives that can be prolonged need or ought to be prolonged?

In the present chapter, I shall be setting the scene for my subsequent arguments for the rejection of the sanctity-of-life view. In Section 1.2, I shall systematize the discussion and arrive, at the end of

[5] World Medical Association, Declaration of Geneva (medical vow adopted by the General Assembly at Geneva, Switzerland, September 1948, and amended by the 22nd World Medical Assembly, Sydney, Australia, 1968).
[6] As cited in Robert M. Veatch: *Case Studies in Medical Ethics* (Cambridge, Mass.: Harvard University Press, 1977), 36.

that section, at the Sanctity-of-Life Principle. This principle states explicitly what is implicit in the view that human life has 'sanctity': that it is absolutely prohibited intentionally to terminate life because all human life, irrespective of its quality or kind, is equally valuable and inviolable.

In Section 1.3, I raise the question as to what makes the taking of human life wrong. The answer that emerges in the context of the sanctity-of-life view seems inadequate, but a short historical digression in Section 1.4 may explain how this view came to be adopted.

In Section 1.5, I give some examples of a common medical practice: to let certain patients die by withholding readily available life-prolonging means. Such practices, supporters of the sanctity-of-life view claim, can be combined with the Sanctity-of-Life Principle. This brings me to the statement of the *qualified* Sanctity-of-Life Principle. This principle holds that whilst it is always absolutely prohibited to terminate life intentionally on the basis of quality-of-life consider-ations, it is sometimes permissible to refrain from preventing death and to let a patient die.

Finally, in Section 1.6, I posit a minimal requirement for ethical argument: consistency. Those supporting the qualified Sanctity-of-Life Principle, I shall argue in Chapters 2, 3, and 4, are—in the absence of a plausible theory of the intentional—prima facie inconsistent because they both prohibit and condone the intentional termination of life, and are typically doing so on the basis of covert quality-of-life considerations.

## 1.2 THE INVIOLABILITY AND EQUAL VALUE OF HUMAN LIFE

The view that all human life is equally valuable and inviolable is deeply rooted in our society. It is enshrined in the law and is at the heart of professional precepts informing the practice of medicine.

The following description of an actual case will serve as an example of the application of the 'sanctity-of-life' view. In May 1981, severely deformed Siamese twins were born in Danville, Illinois. The twins shared a lower body, intestinal tract, and had three legs between them—one normal leg each, and a fused leg with too many toes. Both had trouble breathing and they had to be fed intravenously. The parents and their doctor decided that the twins should be allowed to die. However, against expectations, the twins did not die when medical treatment was withdrawn. When nourishment was withheld, an anonymous telephone caller alerted authorities, and the parents and their doctor were subsequently charged with conspiracy to commit murder. While the Illinois state attorney acknowledged that everyone may have acted from the best of motives when deciding that the infants should be allowed to die, he held:

Motive has nothing to do with it. Quality of life has nothing to do with it. Under no circumstances do you take life because you disagree with the quality of it. These kids have lived and are living human beings. They are entitled to life as long as nature gives it to them.[7]

When awarding custody of the twins to the Family Service Bureau, the Judge agreed that he felt compassion for all involved, but also stated that it was not up to the juvenile court to make philosophical judgements:

The juvenile court must follow the Constitutions of Illinois and the United States, each of which contains a bill of rights. These bills of rights give even to newborn Siamese twins with severe abnormalities an inalienable right to live.[8]

In this case two severely handicapped infants were kept alive against the wishes of their parents, at great expense, and most importantly—irrespective of the infants' prospects to ever lead independent and minimally satisfying lives.[9] If rulings such as these appear to be intolerable because quite oblivious to the interests of all concerned, they are consistent with the sanctity-of-life doctrine's two fundamental tenets: the inviolability of all human life, and the equal value of all human life. Let us take these two notions in turn.

### The Inviolability of Human Life

As far as the inviolability of human life is concerned, the sanctity-of-life doctrine is absolute. The taking of human life, even for reasons of mercy, is not only absolutely prohibited by the law, but also by a medical tradition that can be traced back to the fourth century BC, when doctors first took the Oath of Hippocrates and swore to 'neither give a deadly drug to anyone if asked for it, nor make . . . a suggestion

---

[7] News item, *Independent Journal* (USA), 13 June 1981.

[8] Jeff Lyon: *Playing God in the Nursery* (New York: Norton, 1985), 190.

[9] For a more detailed discussion of the case, see John A. Robertson: 'Dilemma in Danville', *The Hastings Center Report* 11 (1981), 5–8.

to this effect'.[10] Today many doctors and their medical associations regard mercy killing as 'contrary to that for which the medical profession stands'[11] and the law and traditional moral theology regard mercy killing as murder.

Here we should note the following: when speaking of the sanctity-of-life doctrine as absolute, I am not suggesting that the prohibition against the taking of human life has always been held in a universal form, for this would imply total pacifism, and exclude capital punishment and killing in self-defence—practices which are not always condemned by supporters of the sanctity-of-life doctrine. What the sanctity-of-life doctrine prohibits is the intentional termination of *innocent* human life. It is thus, according to the doctrine, not always wrong to kill, but always wrong intentionally to kill an innocent human being. Since the patient is, in the doctor–patient relationship always deemed innocent, natural law theory—one of the corner stones of Catholic moral theology—concurs with the Hippocratic tradition that absolutely prohibits the taking of a patient's life.[12] As the Roman Catholic Church puts it in its *Declaration on Euthanasia*:

It is necessary to state firmly once more that nothing and no one can in any way permit the killing of an innocent human being, whether a foetus or an embryo, an infant or an adult, an old person, or one suffering from an incurable disease, or a person who is dying.[13]

But a further qualification regarding the absolute prohibition of taking life is required. Since there will always be situations where even an absolutist cannot avoid bringing about the death of another person, any absolute prohibition like that of killing must be restricted to what people *intentionally do* to each other. There could, for example, not be an absolute prohibition against ever being responsible for the death of an innocent human being, as an example by the

[10] Quoted from the English translation by Ludwig Edelstein, reprinted in O. Temkin and C. L. Temkin (eds.): *Ancient Medicine: Selected Papers of Ludwig Edelstein* (Baltimore: Johns Hopkins University Press, 1967), 6.

[11] The quotation is from the 1973 Policy Statement of the American Medical Association, as cited by James Rachels: *The End of Life* (Oxford: Oxford University Press, 1986), 88. The AMA's more recent statement of 15 Mar. 1986 reaffirms that the doctor 'should not intentionally cause death'.

[12] There are problems with the natural law position, which prohibits the intentional termination of innocent human lives, but allows for capital punishment and killing in self-defence. I will touch on some of these problems in Ch. 3, Sect. 3.3.

[13] Sacred Congregation for the Doctrine of the Faith: *Declaration on Euthanasia* (Vatican City, 1980), 7.

philosopher Philippa Foot demonstrates. In this case, the brakes of a tram have failed and the driver has a choice of either staying on the present track (thus killing five), or turning the tram onto another track (thereby killing the one person on that track). Whatever the driver does, there will either be one death or five deaths.[14] If the absolute prohibition were to include the prohibition of anything that could result in the death of some innocent person, then it could be obeyed—if at all—only by complete inaction. The sanctity-of-life doctrine thus prohibits *doing* certain things to people, rather than bringing about certain results; it requires that we avoid *intentionally taking* life at all costs, not that we prevent death at all costs. This gives rise to principle *P*1:

> *P*1:  *It is absolutely prohibited intentionally to kill a patient.*

Whilst it is, however, generally true that killing involves us in *doing* something, such as giving a lethal injection, it is also true that we can intentionally bring about death by doing nothing, such as failing to provide a handicapped newborn infant with nourishment and starving it to death. More generally, there are two ways in which we can bring about death: one is to do something which results in someone's death; the other is to fail to do something, the result of which is that someone will die.

Indeed, the Vatican's *Declaration on Euthanasia* defines 'mercy killing' as 'an act or an omission which of itself or by intention causes death',[15] and legal definitions of 'murder' typically include reference to omissions as well as to positive acts. The New South Wales (Australia) Crimes Act, for example, states:

Murder shall be taken to have been committed where the act of the accused, or the thing by him omitted to be done, causing the death charged, was done or omitted with reckless indifference to human life, or with intent to kill or inflict grievous bodily harm upon some person . . .[16]

In the light of the above, principle *P*1 needs to be replaced by principle *P*2:

> *P*2:  *It is absolutely prohibited either intentionally to kill a patient or intentionally to let a patient die.*

[14] Philippa Foot: 'The Problem of Abortion and the Doctrine of Double Effect', in Bonnie Steinbock (ed.): *Killing and Letting Die* (Englewood Cliffs, N.J.: Prentice Hall, 1980), 159.

[15] Op. cit., 6.

[16] The New South Wales (Australia) Crimes Act 1900, S.19 (1)(a).

## The Equal Value of Human Life

If the sanctity-of-life doctrine as it underlies the practice of medicine is absolute in the above sense, it follows that it is absolute in another sense as well: by prohibiting absolutely the intentional termination of *any* human life, it must also absolutely exclude either quality or kind of life as morally relevant factors when deciding whether or not to prolong a patient's life. On this view, all human lives are equal and worthy of the same protection, irrespective of their quality or kind. This point was forcefully made by the Illinois state attorney when commenting on the parents' decision to let their severely handicapped Siamese twins die;[17] it was also confirmed, in 1976, by the Law and Ethics Working Group of the Centre for the Analysis of Health Practices at the Harvard School of Public Health who held that

[b]oth as a standard of medical care and as a statement of philosophy, it is the general policy of hospitals to act affirmatively to preserve the lives of all patients, including persons who suffer from irreversible terminal illness. It is essential that all hospital staff understand this policy and act accordingly.[18]

And in May 1982, the American Department of Health and Human Services issued a 'Notice to Health Care Providers', informing them that, under Section 504 of the Rehabilitation Act, they ran the risk of losing federal funding if handicapped infants were treated differently from normal infants on account of their being handicapped. This notice was followed up with the so-called 'Baby Doe Regulations' which, again, confirmed the Reagan administration's intention to enforce the equal value of all infants' lives. While the 'Baby Doe Regulations' were ultimately quashed in the federal courts, a third response was formulated in Congress as an amendment to the Child Abuse Prevention and Treatment Act, which—while no longer quite as rigid as the 'Baby Doe Regulations'—still stipulates that 'Considerations such as anticipated or actual limited potential of an individual . . . are irrelevant and must not determine the decisions concerning medical care.'[19]

[17] *Independent Journal* (USA), 13 June 1981.

[18] Mitchell T. Rabkin *et al.*: 'Orders Not to Resuscitate', *The New England Journal of Medicine* 295 (1976), 364.

[19] 45CFR Part 1340: Child Abuse and Neglect Prevention and Treatment Program; Proposed Rule, *Federal Register* 49 (238), 48160. For a discussion of the 'Baby Doe Case', see Helga Kuhse and Peter Singer: *Should the Baby Live? The Problem of Handicapped Infants* (Oxford: Oxford University Press, 1985), Ch. 2.

In requiring that all infants—irrespective of their present or future quality of life—be treated equally, the Reagan administration affirmed a fundamental tenet of Anglo-American law. As Sanford Kadish puts it, before the law

all human lives must be regarded as having an equal claim to preservation simply because life is an irreducible value. Therefore, the value of a particular life, over and above the value of life itself, may not be taken into account.[20]

In a recent Australian case also, Mr Justice Vincent, a judge of the Supreme Court, seems to have interpreted the law in this way. Commenting on the case of a baby born with spina bifida who, it was claimed, had been denied life-sustaining treatment, he stressed that 'the law does not permit decisions to be made concerning the quality of life nor any assessment of the value of any human being'.[21]

But if human life constitutes an 'irreducible value', and if the quality or kind of a particular life may not be taken into account when making life or death decisions, then it follows that the *same* effort must go into prolonging one life as goes into prolonging another—even if one patient is irreversibly comatose and the other has a good chance of recovery. At the extreme, this means that we must always do everything possible to prolong life—even if it were decided that a particular patient would be 'better off dead'. At least one physician has interpreted the sanctity-of-life doctrine in this way. David A. Karnofsky, a famous cancer specialist, wrote: 'The patient entrusts his life to his doctor, and it is the doctor's duty to sustain it as long as possible. There should be no suggestion that it is possible for the doctor to do otherwise, even if it were decided that the patient were "better off dead"'.[22]

This attitude, whilst it may strike many of us as cruel and impervious to the interests of the patient, is consistent with the sanctity-of-life doctrine, which absolutely prohibits the intentional termination of any human life, and which thereby also absolutely excludes quality-of-life considerations as a basis for decision-making as far as the prolongation or shortening of human life is concerned.

Whilst the exclusion of quality-of-life considerations is already

[20] Sanford H. Kadish: 'Respect for Life and Regard for Rights in the Criminal Law', in Barker (ed.): *Respect for Life in Medicine*, 72.

[21] *The Age* (Melbourne) 3 July 1986.

[22] D. A. Karnofsky: 'Why Prolong the Life of a Patient with Advanced Cancer?', *Cancer Journal for Clinicians* 10 (1960), 9, as cited by J. B. Wilson: *Death by Decision* (Philadelphia: Westminster Press, 1975), 118.

implied by principle *P*2, principle *P*3 will make this important implication explicit:

*P*3: *It is absolutely prohibited to base decisions relating to the prolongation or shortening of human life on considerations of its quality or kind.*

There is considerable merit in making the exclusion of quality-of-life considerations explicit in this way. Firstly, there are some troubling philosophical difficulties connected with the view that quality or kind of life is morally irrelevant (see Sects. 1.3 and 1.4); and secondly, as we shall see in Chapter 4, the life and death judgements of those supposedly subscribing to the sanctity-of-life view are typically based on the quality or kind of life in question.

If we now conjoin *P*2 and *P*3, we shall have explicated the prohibitory scope of the sanctity-of-life doctrine and have captured what I want to call the 'Sanctity-of-Life Principle' (SLP):

SLP: *It is absolutely prohibited either intentionally to kill a patient or intentionally to let a patient die, and to base decisions relating to the prolongation or shortening of human life on considerations of its quality or kind.*

Now that we have established the prohibitory scope of the sanctity-of-life view, we must ask the question of interest from the ethical perspective: What is it that makes prohibited acts of terminating life wrong?

## 1.3   WHAT'S WRONG WITH TAKING LIFE?

There are a number of possible lines of reply to the question posed in the heading of this section—some religiously inspired, others not. One common claim as to what makes the taking of human life wrong is that an authority, such as God, says it is.

In the development of Western ethical thinking, the appeal to authority has been widespread. Historically, such claims have often been made on behalf of two types of authority: religious teachings, or social practices. Since I believe, however, that G. E. Moore, R. M. Hare, and others have shown conclusively that appeal to authority—as a form of (super)naturalism—is not a defensible ethical position,[23]

[23] G. E. Moore: *Principia Ethica* (Cambridge: Cambridge University Press, 1978), chs. 1, 4; Hare's basic position and opposition to (super)naturalism is put forward in *The Language of Morals* (London: Oxford University Press, 1952), ch. 5; and more recently in *Moral Thinking* (Oxford: Clarendon Press, 1981), ch. 4.

I shall set aside any theistic accounts as to why it is wrong to terminate human life.[24]

Nor do I take the claim to be adequate that there are certain kinds of action (such as killing the innocent) that are wrong 'simply in virtue of their description as such and such identifiable kinds of action'.[25] To take this view may well amount to having opted out of moral thinking altogether, as Jonathan Bennett so forcefully argues.[26]

A more plausible reply seems to be that the taking of human life is wrong because human life is valuable. And, indeed, as we have seen, the sanctity-of-life tradition regards human life not only as inviolable but also as valuable. The Vatican's *Declaration on Euthanasia* discusses the prohibition of euthanasia and suicide under the heading 'The Value of Human Life',[27] and Chief Rabbi Jakobovits captures one important theme of the sanctity-of-life tradition when he attributes an infinite value to human life:

The basic reasoning behind the firm opposition of Judaism to any form of euthanasia proper is the attribution of *infinite* value to every human life. Since infinity is, by definition, indivisible, it follows that every fraction of life, however small, remains equally infinite so that it makes morally no difference whether one shortens life by seventy years or by only a few hours, or whether the victim of murder was young and robust or aged and physically or mentally debilitated.[28]

Dr Moshe Tendler, a professor of Talmudic law, confirms this position:

human life is of infinite value. This in turn means that a piece of infinity is also infinity, and a person who has but a few moments to live is no less of value than a person who has 60 years to live . . . a handicapped individual is a perfect specimen when viewed in an ethical context. The value is an absolute

[24] See Helga Kuhse: 'An Ethical Approach to IVF and ET: What Ethics is All About', in W. Walters and P. Singer (eds.): *Test-tube Babies* (Melbourne: Oxford University Press, 1982), 22–35.

[25] G. E. M. Anscombe: 'Modern Moral Philosophy', *Philosophy* 33 (1958), 10.

[26] Jonathan Bennett: 'Whatever the Consequences', in J. J. Thomson and G. Dworkin (eds.): *Ethics* (New York: Harper & Row, 1968). (The article appeared initially in *Analysis* 26 (1966), 83–102.)

[27] Sacred Congregation: *Declaration on Euthanasia*, 5–6.

[28] Cited by Cardinal John Heenan: Archbishop of Westminster: 'A Fascinating Story', in S. Lack and R. Lamerton (eds.): *The Hour of Our Death: A Record of the Conference on the Care of the Dying held in London in 1973* (London: Chapman, 1974), p. 7.

value. It is not relative to life expectancy, to state of health, or to usefulness to society.[29]

The Protestant theologian Paul Ramsey, professor of religion at Princeton University, takes a similar view:

there is no reason for saying that [six months in the life of a baby born with the invariably fatal Tay-Sachs disease] are a life span of lesser worth to God than living seventy years before the onset of irreversible degeneration. A genuine humanism would say the same thing in other language. It is only a reductive naturalism or social utilitarianism that would regard those months of infant life as worthless because they lead to nothing on a time line of earthly achievements. All our days and years are of equal worth whatever the consequence; death is not more a tragedy at one time than another.[30]

And if these theistic accounts appear to put an absolute value on human life, so does secular legal theory—at least as far as the practice of medicine is concerned. As Edward Keyserlingk puts it in his study written for the Law Reform Commission of Canada: *Sanctity of Life or Quality of Life*:

in the medical arena, when decisions about life and death and the integrity of life are directly at issue, legal theory appears to consider sanctity of life not just *one* factor among others in determining prohibitions, responsibilities and sanctions—it is the conclusive and fundamental factor.[31]

However, whilst the reply that the taking of human life is wrong because human life has sanctity, or is (infinitely) valuable, has an initial plausibility, it will not do because it comes close to being tautological: it simply asserts that there is value in what the taking of life takes away. A more plausible reply as to what makes the taking of human life wrong would be this one: it is wrong to take human life because human life is life of a very special kind. What makes it wrong to take life is thus the fact, if it is a fact, that *human* life is absolutely valuable.

But this reply is, again, less than satisfactory because we may ask what it is that gives special significance to life that is human. Here it will not do to answer that human life has sanctity because it takes the form of a featherless biped, or because it can be identified as belonging to the species *Homo sapiens*. In other words, the wrongness

---

[29] Cited by Howard Brody: *Ethical Discussions in Medicine* (Boston: Little, Brown, 1976), 66.

[30] Paul Ramsey: *Ethics at the Edges of Life* (New Haven: Yale University Press, 1978), 191.

[31] Keyserlingk: *Sanctity of Life or Quality of Life*, 3–4.

of taking human life must not rest on what has come to be known as 'speciesism' (a notion I shall discuss more fully in Chapter 5)—namely, the view that is is morally justifiable to treat human life differently from other relevantly similar non-human life, simply because it is human.[32]

Rather, an acceptable reply would have to make reference to some essentially human characteristic or characteristics, other than that it is merely bodily human life, such as consciousness, or the ability to experience pleasurable states. If this were the reply, then it would follow that also some non-human animal life has sanctity and should be respected.

Or the reply might be, human life has sanctity because human beings are rational, purposeful moral beings, with hopes, ambitions, preferences, life-purposes, ideals, and so on. While the characteristics mentioned here will vary with the ethical theory one espouses, what is clear, though, is this: if one takes the present approach, then one is not saying that human life, *qua* human life, has sanctity, but rather that rationality, the satisfaction of preferences, the holding of ideals, and so on, has sanctity. Of course, one may still hold that it is wrong to take human life, but only insofar as human life is a precondition for the existence of rationality, the experiencing of pleasurable states, or whatever else one takes the valuable characteristic to be. But if one takes this view, then it would be difficult to argue that it would be wrong, even prima facie, to terminate the lives of the irreversibly comatose, or the lives of those who do not possess and never will possess any of the characteristic(s) taken to be valuable.[33]

That, however, is not the view underlying the sanctity-of-life tradition. In the sanctity-of-life tradition, all human lives are of the same value and have an equal claim to protection, irrespective of their quality or kind. In other words, human life is not regarded as a means to a further end (such as consciousness, rationality, and so on), but as an intrinsic good. To adopt the language of traditional moralists, bodily human life is not a *bonum utile*, or useful good, but rather a *bonum honestum*, that is, a good in itself.[34] As Sanford H. Kadish puts it in the previously cited quotation: 'life is an irreducible value.

---

[32] See Peter Singer: *Practical Ethics* (Cambridge: Cambridge University Press, 1979), esp. ch. 4.

[33] See Frankena: 'Ethics of Respect for Life', 50–4.

[34] See William May: 'Ethics and Human Identity: The Challenge of the New Biology', *Horizons* 3 (1976), 35, for a critique of the approach that life is merely a *bonum utile*.

Therefore, the value of a particular life, over and above the value of life itself, may not be taken into account.'[35] Or, again, as it is stated in the Vatican's *Declaration on Euthanasia* 'nothing and no one can in any way permit the killing of an innocent human being, whether a foetus or an embryo, an infant or an adult, an old person, or one suffering from an incurable disease, or a person who is dying'.[36]

The position is summed up by the biologist Jean Rostand, when she writes: 'there is no life so degraded, debased, deteriorated, or impoverished that it does not deserve respect and is not worth defending with zeal and conviction'.[37]

But the view that bodily human life is a basic, intrinsic good, even if accepted, is insufficient to support the full sanctity-of-life view, which sees the taking of human life as *always* wrong. Let us, for the moment, accept that mere bodily human life is a basic or intrinsic good. But even if we accept that proposition, it is of course not clear how supporters of the sanctity-of-life view can derive an absolute prohibition of the intentional termination of life from this. All that is entailed by the proposition that human life is a good in itself is that it is prima facie wrong to take human life—not that it is always and absolutely wrong. For if life is a basic and intrinsic good, what objection could there be to intentionally taking one life in order to save two? The absolute prohibition of the intentional termination of life, rather than its prima facie wrongness, must come from somewhere else. And so it does. As we shall see in the next section, the absolute prohibition of the intentional termination of life has its source in theology, and makes but little sense outside that particular framework.

Moreover, if, according to the sanctity-of-life doctrine, mere human life is intrinsically valuable, and if the wrongness of terminating life consists in taking away what has value, then this is not only a theoretically unconvincing position, it is also one that has unacceptable practical consequences. On the sanctity-of-life view, it would, for example, be just as wrong to terminate the life of a permanently comatose patient as it would be to take the life of a conscious or self-conscious human being. Similarly, the fact that a patient is dying from cancer and is suffering excruciating pain would not, in itself, be

---

[35] Kadish: 'Respect for Life', 72.

[36] Op. cit., 7.

[37] Jean Rostand: *Humanly Possible: A Biologist's Notes on the Future of Mankind* (New York: Saturday Review Press, 1973), as cited by Keyserlingk: *Sanctity of Life or Quality of Life*, 21–2.

a reason for refraining from resuscitating her were she to suffer a heart attack. On the sanctity-of-life view, it seems, a patient's life would have to be prolonged even if continued life were not a good to her—or to anyone else. Those who take the view that life can cease to be a good would simply be mistaken.

Whilst, as we shall see, doctors and those subscribing to the sanctity-of-life doctrine do not always consistently apply the principle that all bodily human life is equally valuable and inviolable, the sanctity-of-life doctrine is the theoretical bedrock of medical ethics and the law. If the doctrine strikes many of us as highly implausible, a short historical digression may help to explain how it came to be adopted.

### 1.4   A HISTORICAL DIGRESSION

Every society known to us subscribes to some principle or principles involving respect for human life. As Georgia Harkness puts it:

In every society there appears to be an elemental reverence for life which makes the deliberate killing of another person a punishable offence. In all societies there are exceptions . . . yet aversion to murder is probably the most universal of all moral attitudes.[38]

But if aversion to murder, or wrongful killing, is universal, there have been great variations between cultural traditions as to what constitutes *wrongful* killing.

If we turn to the roots of our Western tradition, we find that in Greek and Roman times not all human life was regarded as inviolable and worthy of protection. Slaves and 'barbarians' did not have a full right to life, and human sacrifices and gladiatorial combat were acceptable at different times. Spartan law required that deformed infants be put to death;[39] for Plato, infanticide is one of the regular institutions of the ideal state;[40] Aristotle regards abortion as a desirable option;[41] and the Stoic philosopher Seneca writes unapolo-

[38] Georgia Harkness: *The Sources of Western Morality* (New York: Charles Scribner's Sons, 1954), 24.
[39] See James Rachels: 'Euthanasia', in Tom Regan (ed.): *Matters of Life and Death* (New York: Random House, 1980), 32.
[40] Plato: *Republic* trans. H. D. P. Lee, bk v, sect. 460 (Harmondsworth: Penguin, 1972), 216.
[41] Aristotle: 'Politics', bk vii, sect. 1335, in R. McKeon (ed.): *The Basic Works of Aristotle* (New York: Random House, 1941), 1302.

getically: 'unnatural progeny we destroy; we drown even children who at birth are weakly and abnormal'.[42]

Stoic and Epicurean philosophers thought that suicide and euthanasia were acceptable options when life no longer held any value. Once again to quote Seneca:

I shall not abandon old age, if old age preserves me intact as regards the better part of myself; but if old age begins to shatter my mind, and to pull its various faculties to pieces, if it leaves me, not life, but only the breath of life, I shall rush out of a house that is crumbling and tottering. I shall not avoid illness by seeking death, as long as the illness is curable and does not impede my soul. I shall not lay violent hands upon myself just because I am in pain; for death under such circumstances is defeat. But if I find out that the pain must always be endured, I shall depart, not because of the pain, but because it will be a hindrance to me as regards all my reasons for living.[43]

And whilst there were deviations from these views (one of which is the Hippocratic Oath, briefly to be discussed below), it is probably correct to say that such practices as abortion, infanticide, suicide, and euthanasia were less proscribed in ancient times than they are today. There has been a gradual expansion of the circle protecting human life, outlawing not only the killing of slaves or 'barbarians', gladiatorial combat, and human sacrifice, but also abortion, infanticide, and euthanasia.

Most historians of Western morals agree that the rise of Judaism and even more of Christianity contributed greatly to the general feeling that human life is valuable and worthy of respect.

W. E. H. Lecky gives the now classical account of the sanctity of human life in his *History of European Morals*:

Considered as immortal beings, destined for the extremes of happiness or of misery, and united to one another by a special community of redemption, the first and most manifest duty of the Christian man was to look upon his fellowmen as sacred beings and from this notion grew up the eminently Christian idea of the sanctity of human life . . . it was one of the most important services of Christianity that besides quickening greatly our benevolent affections it definitely and dogmatically asserted the sinfulness of all destruction of human life as a matter of amusement, or of simple convenience, and thereby formed a new standard higher than any which then existed in the world . . . This minute and scrupulous care for human life and

---

[42] Seneca 'De Ira', trans. J. W. Basure, in T. E. Page *et al.* (eds.): *Seneca Moral Essays*, vol. i (London: Heinemann, 1961), 409.
[43] Seneca: '58th Letter to Lucilius', trans. R. M. Gummere, in T. E. Page *et al.* (eds.): *Seneca: Ad Lucilium Epistulae Morales*, vol. i (London: Heinemann, 1961), 409.

virtue in the humblest form, in the slave, the gladiator, the savage, or the infant, was indeed wholly foreign to the genius of Paganism. It was produced by the Christian doctrine of the inestimable value of each immortal soul.[44]

Whilst it is true that even before the rise of Christianity some philosophical and religious schools expressed a strong respect for human life, it is generally agreed that such views were only held by a minority. For example, the Hippocratic Oath, which Ludwig Edelstein assigns to the fourth century BC, already strongly disapproves of abortion, euthanasia, and suicide—independently of Judaeo-Christian influence. However, if Edelstein is correct, this oath represented only 'a small segment of Greek opinion' and was not generally accepted until the end of antiquity when Christianity became the dominant religion. Edelstein attributes the oath to the Pythagoreans who strongly condemned suicide on the grounds that 'we are all soldiers of God, placed in an appointed post of duty, which it is a rebellion against our Maker to desert'.[45]

Whatever the importance of the Pythagoreans in the evolution of the idea of the sanctity of human life, it would seem that at least one strand of their view, namely, the belief that we must not take our own life because God has assigned a certain post to us, is continued in the more influential Christian tradition (both Catholic and Protestant), which holds that we are God's property and must not quit our station in life wilfully. Life is, in the Christian tradition, not our own to do with as we like, but is 'entirely an ordination, a loan and a stewardship'.[46] From such presuppositions it follows quite logically that 'only God has the right to take the life of an innocent'[47] and that 'man . . . must wait his appointed time till his charge cometh, till he sinks and is crushed with the weight of his own misery'.[48]

On this view, then, it is not human life as such which is inviolable or has sanctity; it is rather the will of God which has sanctity and must

[44] W. E. H. Lecky: *History of European Morals from Augustus to Charlemagne*, 11th edn. (London: Longmans Green & Co., 1894), vol. ii, pp. 18, 20, 34.

[45] Temkin and Temkin (eds.): *Ancient Medicine*, 6, 14 ff.; see also W. E. H. Lecky, *History of European Morals*, vol. ii, pp. 17–61.

[46] Paul Ramsey, as quoted by Daniel Callahan: 'The Sanctity of Life', in Donald R. Cutler (ed.): *Updating Life and Death* (Boston: Beacon Press, 1969), 186; see also Ramsey: *Ethics at the Edges of Life*, 147. A similar view is expressed by Thomas Aquinas in *Summa Theologiae* II, ii, question 64, article 5.

[47] Gerald Kelly: *Medico-moral Problems* (St Louis: Catholic Hospital Association of the United States and Canada, 1958), 5.

[48] Humphrey Primatt: *A Dissertation on the Duty of Mercy and the Sin of Cruelty to Brute Animals* (London, 1776), 65. I owe this reference to James Rachels: 'Euthanasia', 47.

not be violated. As the theologian Karl Barth puts it: 'Life itself does not create this respect. The command of God creates respect for it.'[49] It is thus not killing as such which is wrong, but it is wrong to act contrary to the will of God. In other words, killing is not an act wrong either in itself or wrong because of what it does to the victim; rather, killing is wrong simply because it is contrary to the will of God.

But, according to the sanctity-of-life doctrine, human life is not only inviolable, it is also valuable. Where, then, do those writing in the Christian tradition locate this value? It is often thought that human life is valuable and deserves respect because human beings have immortal souls. W. E. H. Lecky attributes, as we have seen, the Christian's 'minute and scrupulous care for human life' to the 'doctrine of the inestimable value of each immortal soul'. But here we should note that it does not necessarily follow from the belief that each human being has an immortal soul of inestimable value that bodily life as such has value. In this context, it seems quite plausible to hold, for example, that the body is a tomb or prison from which the immortal soul seeks to be set free; and whilst one could try to argue for the unity of body and soul, it would appear that a more plausible answer is provided by the Protestant moral theologian, Paul Ramsey. Ramsey holds that the value of human life 'is ultimately grounded in the value God is placing on it'. In other words, human life has value because God values His creatures. The value is thus, on this view, not *in* human life; it is rather an 'alien' value, bestowed by God on each human being, and not something 'inherent in man'.[50] Human life does not have intrinsic value (nor is it valuable because those possessing it value it); rather, it derives its value from an extrinsic source: God. This means that the taking of human life is wrong only in so far as it is contrary to the 'Thou shalt not' entailed by the divine valuation of human life.

Such accounts of the sanctity of human life thus rest on the view that ethics consists in conformity with the will of God, there being nothing intrinsically right or wrong about terminating or not prolonging human life, nothing sacred in itself about human life. Moreover, to the extent that God is the final arbiter of right or wrong, good or bad, His commands must be obeyed without exception— they are absolute.

[49] Karl Barth: *Church Dogmatics* vol. 3 (Edinburgh: Clark, 1961), part 4. 339.
[50] Paul Ramsey: 'The Morality of Abortion', in D. L. Labby (ed.): *Life or Death* (Seattle: University of Washington Press, 1968), 72–4.

There is no longer a universal acceptance of religion and of the belief that ethics consists in doing what God commands. Conventional attitudes based on these beliefs are, however, still very much with us today. During the long period when Christian beliefs moulded European thought, the sanctity-of-life view became part of an unquestioned moral tradition: it became part of medical ethics and the law. It was, for example, not until 1516 that Sir Thomas More presented the first important defence of mercy killing in the Christian era,[51] and it was not until the seventeenth and eighteenth centuries that philosophers began to question the view that ethics requires a religious basis. From such initial philosophical questionings, however, it is a long way to a fundamental change in popular attitudes. Whilst it is today no longer generally believed that life has sanctity in the religious sense, the ethical attitudes to which these religious beliefs gave rise still find expression in the deep-seated belief that human life, irrespective of its quality or kind, is absolutely inviolable and equally valuable; and that we must never take life—either our own or that of anyone else—because life is not *ours* to do with as we see fit.

But now we must be clear about just what a non-theistic account of the sanctity of human life entails. While it may have made some religious sense to hold that mere bodily life has sanctity because life is a gift from God and has received its value from Him, it makes but poor philosophical sense to say that mere bodily life is intrinsically valuable and absolutely inviolable—for a secular account of the sanctity of human life will be hard put to provide a convincing reason for this view. As we have already noted above, to assert that terminating or not prolonging life is wrong because the state of being alive is itself intrinsically valuable barely rises to the level of an argument for the inviolability of human life. It simply asserts that there is value in what we fail to preserve or in what the taking of life takes away. What possible reason could there be for holding that it is intrinsically wrong to terminate the life of a permanently comatose patient? What could be a possible reason for holding that it is intrinsically wrong to refrain from prolonging the life of an infant so seriously handicapped that it will experience only pain and suffering, making its existence 'worse than nothing'?

The point is this. A secular account of the sanctity-of-life view will be highly implausible to all those who see human life not as a good in

[51] Thomas More: *Utopia*, bk. ii (Cambridge: Cambridge University Press, 1908), 122.

itself, but rather as a precondition for 'something else'; it will be an unattractive position to all those who, for example, see life in a permanent coma as in no way preferable to death.[52] In short, for most of us it is not mere life that is valuable, it is rather that we value those things that life makes possible. This point is made by the utilitarian philosopher Henry Sidgwick who, in arguing against Herbert Spencer, describes the function of morality as consisting

in maintaining such habits and sentiments as are necessary to the continued existence, in full numbers, of a society of human beings . . . But this is not because the mere existence of human organisms, even if prolonged to eternity, appears to me in any way desirable; it is only assumed to be so because it is supposed to be accompanied by Consciousness on the whole desirable; it is therefore this Desirable Consciousness which we must regard as ultimate Good.[53]

Whether or not 'Desirable Consciousness' is the ultimate good is not our present concern—although I shall be raising this and related issues in Chapter 5. What is clear, though, is that those who subscribe to the sanctity-of-life view are not impervious to the arguments put forward by Henry Sidgwick and his fellow utilitarians. But to the extent that supporters of the sanctity-of-life doctrine pay heed to consequentialist considerations, such as states of consciousness, they are abandoning their pure absolutist stance. And an impure Absolutism does, as we shall see, face some very serious problems.

## 1.5   THOU SHALT NOT KILL; BUT NEED'ST NOT STRIVE OFFICIOUSLY TO KEEP ALIVE

Many of those in the medical profession who profess to subscribe to the sanctity-of-life doctrine appear not to practise what the doctrine preaches. Each year, thousands of handicapped infants are 'allowed to die',[54] terminally ill patients do not have their lives prolonged by all possible means,[55] and the life-support of irreversibly comatose

---

[52] See also Jonathan Glover: *Causing Death and Saving Lives* (Harmondsworth: Penguin, 1977), 45.

[53] Henry Sidgwick: *The Ethics of T. H. Green, H. Spencer, and J. Martineau* (London: Macmillan, 1902), 144.

[54] *New York Times* 16 June 1974. I owe this reference to Singer: *Practical Ethics*, 229.

[55] See, e.g., James Rachels: 'Euthanasia, Killing and Letting Die', in John Ladd (ed.): *Ethical Issues Relating to Life and Death* (New York: Oxford University Press, 1979), 150, on the practice of 'no coding'.

patients is withdrawn in the clear expectation that death will often follow within minutes.[56] But if lives such as these could be prolonged by readily available means and a decision is taken against prolonging them, then we appear to be confronted with practices that do not treat all lives as equally valuable and inviolable. This is denied by supporters of the sanctity-of-life view, who believe that the absolute Sanctity-of-Life Principle can be combined with a limited duty of life-preservation.

Doctors thus frequently cite the nineteenth-century poet Arthur Clough in support of their practice to let some patients die. Arthur Clough gave currency to the lines which provide the heading to this section:

> 'Thou shalt not kill; but need'st not strive
> Officiously to keep alive.

Somewhat ironically, though, these lines were not meant as the authoritative ethical pronouncement they are often taken to be; rather, they come from the satirical poem *The Latest Decalogue*, which begins with the following lines:

> Thou shalt have one god only; who
> would be at the expense of two.
>
> No graven images may be
> worshipped except the currency.[57]

Thus Arthur Clough himself does not appear to believe that 'not striving to keep alive' is morally somewhat more commendable than killing, but the view that a morally relevant difference exists between killing and at least some instances of letting die is widespread. It is, for example, implied by both the 1973 and 1986 policy statements of the American Medical Association. The 1973 statement begins by condemning the intentional termination of life as contrary to that for which the medical profession stands, and then continues by apparently condoning letting die:

The cessation of the employment of extraordinary means to prolong the life of the body when there is irrefutable evidence that biological death is imminent is the decision of the patient and/or his immediate family. The

---

[56] See, e.g., *70 N.J. 10, In the Matter of Karen Quinlan, an Alleged Incompetent*, Supreme Court of New Jerey, Argued Jan. 26, 1976, Decided March 31, 1976, reprinted in Steinbock (ed.): *Killing and Letting Die*, 23–44.

[57] 'The Latest Decalogue' is included in Helen Gardner (ed.): *The New Oxford Book of English Verse* (Oxford: Oxford University Press, 1978).

advice and judgment of the physician should be freely available to the patient and/or his immediate family.[58]

Similarly the 1986 statement of the Association: it holds that a doctor 'should not intentionally cause death', and then continues to outline the conditions when it is permissible to allow a patient to die.[59]

The same general belief is contained in the Vatican's *Declaration on Euthanasia*,[60] is part of the ethico-legal education of Australian medical students,[61] and is frequently condoned by the law.[62] Our moral and professional codes of conduct thus condemn killing and the intentional termination of life, and condone—and even commend[63]—the practice of letting some patients die. Various grounds are offered by supporters of the sanctity-of-life view as to what makes killing different, or worse, from letting die, and these grounds will be examined in subsequent chapters. Here we should merely note that supporters of the Sanctity-of-Life Principle are widely agreed that whilst killing is always wrong, it is not always wrong for a doctor to refrain from preventing a patient's death.

Those supporters of the Sanctity-of-Life Principle who believe that not all lives that can be prolonged must be prolonged are subscribing to what I have called the *qualified* Sanctity-of-Life-Principle (qSLP):

qSLP: *It is absolutely prohibited either intentionally to kill a patient or intentionally to let a patient die, and to base decisions relating to the prolongation or shortening of human life on considerations of its quality or kind; it is, however, sometimes permissible to refrain from preventing death.*

To be internally consistent, the qSLP clearly must presuppose that refraining from preventing death is not—or at least not always—an instance of the intentional termination of life; in addition to that, the absolute prohibition of the intentional termination of any human life

[58] 1973 Policy Statement of the American Medical Association, as cited by Rachels: *The End of Life*, 88.
[59] The 1986 statement of the AMA's Council on Ethical and Judicial Affairs is dated 15 Mar. 1986. It was distributed by the AMA in typescript form.
[60] Sacred Congregation: *Declaration on Euthanasia*, 9–11.
[61] Arthur W. Burton: *Medical Ethics and the Law* (Glebe: Australasian Medical Publishing Co., 1979), 63.
[62] See, e.g., the recent American 'Baby Doe Case', where a local court in Indiana upheld the parents' decision to let their Down's syndrome infant die by withholding food, water, and surgery. For a discussion of this case see Kuhse and Singer: *Should the Baby Live?*
[63] See the editorial article: 'Doctors "Not Guilty" of Prolonging Life at Any Cost', *Hastings Center Report* 9 (1979), 2–3.

also implies that the principles espoused to distinguish between permissible and impermissible actions, or omissions that result in a foreseen death, must not be based on quality-of-life considerations.

In Chapters 2, 3, and 4, I shall argue that these presuppositions are false. Firstly, I shall attempt to show that the practical judgements of supporters of the qSLP are typically based on quality-of-life considerations. Secondly, in the absence of a coherent theory of intention that allows us to distinguish—in the way supporters of the qSLP want us to distinguish—between prohibited and permissible instances of bringing about death, I shall argue, we must regard all instances of refraining from preventing death as instances of the intentional termination of life. If this is correct, then the qSLP ought to be rejected on the grounds of inconsistency—for it both prohibits and condones the intentional termination of life.

### 1.6   CONSISTENCY AND ETHICS

It is often held that moral disagreement such as that between supporters of a sanctity-of-life view and, say, supporters of a consequentialist quality-of-life ethics, is unsettlable and interminable. Alasdair MacIntyre, for example, has argued that when Thomistic or Kantian notions about an absolute moral law are matched against premises about individual rights and post-Benthamite notions of utility, it will be found that these premises are incommensurable with each other and 'argument characteristically gives way to the increasingly shrill battle of assertion with counter-assertions'.[64]

Similarly the philosopher Philippa Foot: in a well-known article published in 1958, she suggested that ethical debate often breaks down because it depends as much on imagination as on argument in the ordinary sense of the term, where one person may simply be unable to 'see' what the other person is getting at.[65] But even if we accept that Philippa Foot is at least partially right and that questions of ultimate ends may not be amenable to direct proof,[66] this does not mean that ethical debate is altogether impossible. For those unable to 'see', it may be a rewarding experience to abandon at least temporarily the lofty heights of pure theory and to apply one's own

[64] Alasdair MacIntyre: 'Why is the Search for the Foundation of Ethics so Frustrating?', *Hastings Center Report* 9 (1979), 16.

[65] Philippa Foot: 'Moral Arguments', *Mind* 67 (1958), 513.

[66] See also John Stuart Mill: *Utilitarianism* (London: Collins, 1968), 288.

fundamental axioms, and those of others, to concrete situations to see just what they come to in those situations. This may assist where the ordinary philosophical imagination fails. In addition to that, and more importantly, even if ultimate ends are non-rational, reason does still have a major role to play in settling moral disputes. R. M. Hare stresses the importance of rational method in ethical argument[67] and contemporary subjectivists such as J. L. Mackie[68] and J. J. C. Smart[69] agree that even if ethical judgements are non-cognitive and cannot be verified or falsified, arguments in support of moral judgements are nonetheless amenable to solution by rational method.

One point on which probably everyone in the history of ethical thinking has agreed is that ethical judgements must be consistent. Consistency is, of course, not a specifically ethical requirement; rather, it is a formal requirement basic to all minimally rational discourse. Nor is it a sufficient requirement. As R. B. Brandt has put it: 'Perhaps the devil is perfectly consistent, but all his ethical principles are incorrect.'[70] A person could thus act unethically even though she is entirely consistent in following, say, racist or sexist principles. But despite this, the fact remains that reason and consistency are inextricably linked. If consistency is not a sufficient requirement for rationality or for ethical judgements, it is a necessary one. Whatever else reason may be thought to include—and here a list would be both long and heterogeneous—there is no doubt that it would include consistency. If it were thus possible to uncover an internal inconsistency in somebody's ethical views, we could be certain to have dealt them a mortal blow.

This book is about two major inconsistencies in the views of those who subscribe to the qualified Sanctity-of-Life Principle. Supporters of the qSLP, I shall argue, are being inconsistent in at least one, but typically two, respects:

1. In holding that it is in some circumstances permissible to refrain from preventing death, they infringe the previously accepted principle which holds that it is always absolutely prohibited

[67] Hare: *Language of Morals; idem: Moral Thinking; idem: Freedom and Reason* (Oxford: Oxford University Press, 1963).
[68] J. L. Mackie: *Ethics: Inventing Right and Wrong* (Harmondsworth: Penguin, 1977).
[69] J. J. C. Smart: 'An Outline of a System of Utilitarian Ethics', in J. J. C. Smart and Bernard Williams: *Utilitarianism For and Against* (Cambridge: Cambridge University Press, 1973) 3–67.
[70] R. B. Brandt: *Ethical Theory* (Englewood Cliffs, NJ: Prentice Hall, 1959), 18.

    intentionally to terminate life. Refraining from preventing death, I shall argue, is in these circumstances an instance of the intentional termination of life.

2. They affirm the equality of all human lives and yet base their arguments for a limited duty of life-preservation on implicit quality-of-life considerations.

Typically, supporters of the qSLP deny that their judgements are based on quality-of-life considerations, or are instances of the intentional termination of life. Rather, they cite one or more of a number of possible distinctions which, they claim, allow us to differentiate in a morally relevant way between instances of the intentional termination of life and an agent's refraining from preventing death. Examples of such distinctions are those between

—acts and omissions
—causing death and allowing death to occur
—ordinary and extraordinary means of treatment
—intending death and merely foreseeing that death will occur as a
   consequence of the agent's action or omission.

The argument is that these distinctions have moral significance in themselves, irrespective of quality-of-life considerations, and can be employed to show that whilst it would always be wrong intentionally to terminate life, it would not always be wrong to refrain from preserving it.

    I believe it can be shown that none of the more plausible distinctions suggested have moral significance in themselves, and that the only relevant difference between what are regarded as prohibited instances of the intentional termination of life and what are regarded as permissible instances of not prolonging it are quality-of-life or consequentialist considerations. This means that all those who want to combine the pure absolutism of the Sanctity-of-Life Principle with a limited duty of life-preservation are being inconsistent.

    The central argument of this book is thus that the qualified SLP is untenable and ought to be rejected because it is internally inconsistent. This leaves the 'pure' Sanctity-of-Life Principle, untempered by a limited duty of life-preservation. If we were to act in accordance with this principle, medicine would be entering its zealous phase, where the preservation of life would take precedence over all other medical and social objectives. Every wisp of life would have to be preserved, irrespective of whether such measures would be benefiting or harming an individual patient. However, such a position is not only intuitively implausible, it is also ultimately unintelligible.

Absolutist principles presuppose limits, either in terms of the distinction between acts and omissions, or between intended and foreseen consequences. If, as I shall argue, these limits cannot plausibly be drawn, then the pure SLP fails as an action-guiding principle. If an agent is equally responsible for all the foreseen consequences of an action (or an omission), as well as for what she intends, there will be conflict cases where the SLP requires incompatible actions so that the principle cannot be absolute: an agent would be breaking the absolute prohibition against the intentional termination of life, no matter what she does or doesn't do. Hence, since 'ought' implies 'can', one cannot be absolutely obliged to perform two acts (or omissions) of which, as things are, one cannot perform both.[71] This means that the absolute SLP is tenable neither in a qualified nor in an unqualified form.

It is important to see that in adhering to the qualified SLP, we are faced not merely with a theoretically confused doctrine— something of interest only to philosophers and moral theologians—but with a misleading doctrine that has indefensible consequences in practice as well. As will become apparent throughout this book, medical decision-making is frequently based on morally irrelevant grounds, is inconsistent and idiosyncratic, and results in much unnecessary suffering and the wasting of limited resources.

In the light of our growing control over life and death, the sanctity-of-life view becomes increasingly implausible—even at an intuitive level. The point is not only that 'new medicine calls all in doubt'; there is, as the American bioethicist Robert Veatch notes, 'something about the life and death issues raised by advanced medical technology which *forces* us to rethink all the basic problems of morality'.[72] We are forced to rethink many problems of morality because adherence to traditional tenets can often be bought only at the price of increasingly blatant inconsistencies.

These inconsistencies express themselves in the idiosyncratic practices of individual doctors and hospitals, but they have their source in the ultimately untenable views that all human life is absolutely inviolable and equally valuable, and that nevertheless it is

[71] See also Mackie: *Ethics*, 160–8.
[72] As cited by K. L. Woodward: 'The Ethics of Miracles', *Newsweek* 19 Sept. 1977, 57.

sometimes permissible to refrain from preventing a patient's death on the basis of what are implicit and unarticulated quality-of-life considerations. These unreconciled and unreconcilable tenets quite naturally lead to muddled practice: both as regards those quality-of-life criteria that form the basis for life and death decisions, and also as far as the method is concerned by which those life and death decisions are then carried out. The slow and often distressing method of letting die is taken to be morally preferable to helping a patient die, or to killing her.

But, as medical science and technology progresses, inconsistencies in our thoughts and actions are becoming more and more pronounced and can no longer be ignored. 'Cognitive dissonance' forces us to examine critically what we think and what we do. This means that inconsistencies in our beliefs and actions can be motivating factors in their own right—that is, have a profound influence on our ethical views. On this, philosophers from rather different backgrounds are agreed. The German Marxist philosopher Juergen Habermas puts it this way: 'Normative structures can be overturned directly through cognitive dissonance between secular knowledge—expanded with the development of the forces of production—and the dogmatics of traditional world views.'[73]

Peter Singer, writing in the post-Benthamite British tradition, makes the same point, although in somewhat less convoluted prose: 'if we sense an inconsistency in our beliefs and actions, we will try to do something to eliminate the sense of inconsistency, just as when we feel hungry we will try to do someting to eliminate our hunger'. One way of doing this, Peter Singer continues, is to make 'our beliefs and actions both true and consistent'.[74]

As regards our present concern, the quest for consistency must involve a critical examination of the sanctity-of-life doctrine's two basic tenets: the absolute inviolability of human life, and the equal value of all human life. This book is a contribution towards such a critical examination. In common with all critiques, my approach is largely negative and destructive, rather than constructive: I am concerned to show that, and why, the qualified SLP will not do—that

[73] Juergen Habermas: *Legitimation Crisis*, trans. T. McCarthy (Boston: Beacon Press, 1975), 12. For one of the seminal psychological works on cognitive dissonance, see Leon Festinger: *A Theory of Cognitive Dissonance* (Stanford: Stanford University Press, 1957).

[74] Peter Singer: *The Expanding Circle* (New York: Farrar, Straus & Giroux, 1981), 143.

it is a muddled principle which has unacceptable practical consequences.

But if I am successful in this, I shall also be constructive in Singer's
and Habermas's sense—namely in adding to, or creating, 'cognitive
dissonance', and in thus helping to clear the way for a new look at the
practice of medicine and the moral dilemmas raised by its revolution-
ary advances. Such a new look, I suggest, can no longer ignore
quality-of-life considerations; but to accept that the quality or kind of
a patient's life can ever be morally relevant reason as to whether she
should live or die is to abandon the sanctity-of-life view and to accept
a quality-of-life ethics instead. I shall provide a sketch of such a
quality-of-life ethics in Chapter 5.

Here we return to the beginning. The Copernican Revolution
meant not only that the earth had lost its central position in the
universe, but also that the Great Chain of Being had been broken
once and for all. As John Donne puts it, with the sun lost and the
cosmos 'all in pieces', 'Prince, Subject, Father, Son are things forgot'.
And just as Thomas Hobbes and John Locke were compelled to work
out anew the meanings of authority and subjection, so shall we, faced
with a revolution in the biomedical sciences, have to work out anew
the meanings of life and death, what it is that gives special value to
human life, and when (and for whom) death is an evil.

The uncritical retention of the Sanctity-of-Life Principle is consti-
tutive of what Socrates called the 'unexamined life', which he
regarded as no life for a human being. How can we examine our lives
and practices? Through rational discourse and argumentation. As
Juergen Habermas puts it—and as almost every philosopher will
agree—once called into question, truth claims can be resolved only
through the force of the better argument, through an analysis of the
notion of providing rational grounds.[75] And such grounds, I suggest
in Chapter 5, will ineluctably include quality-of-life criteria.

To begin, then, I want to investigate the traditional view that a
distinction—both in terms of causal efficacy and in terms of moral
responsibility—can be drawn between our deliberate actions and our
deliberate omissions; or, to put it in terms relevant for our
investigations, between killing and letting die.

---

[75] Habermas: *Legitimation Crisis*, part iii.

# 2

# Causing Death
# and Not Prolonging Life

Thou shalt have one God only; who
Would be at the expense of two?
No graven images may be
Worshipped, except the currency.
. . . Thou shalt not kill, but needst not strive
Officiously to keep alive. . . .

A. H. Clough: 'The Latest Decalogue'

*Cohen*: . . . Supposing you have a child born physically apparently well, but virtually an ament. I am sure you would say that child must remain alive; so you would differentiate, as it were, between the omission of means of saving life, and the commission of means of destroying life. Am I right in that? *Miller*: Yes. In other words, I don't think there's any point in operating on a congenital heart defect in a Mongolian idiot, on the other hand, there is no excuse for going around slaughtering healthy Mongols. *Cohen*: I think this really comes down, doesn't it, to A. H. Clough's observation, 'Thou shalt not kill, but needst not strive officiously to keep alive.' I think most doctors would follow that doctrine, don't you? *Miller*: Yes.

> *From*: 'Keeping People Alive', in A. Clow (ed.): *Morals and Medicine*, as cited by Glover: *Causing Death and Saving Lives*, p. 152

'And let me tell you this, too, Mother: everyone of us is responsible for everyone else in every way, and I most of all.' Mother could not help smiling at that. She wept and smiled at the same time. 'How are you', she said, 'most of all responsible for everyone? There are murderers and robbers in the world, and what terrible sin have you committed that you should accuse yourself before everyone else?' 'Mother, my dearest heart,' he said, (he had begun using such caressing, such unexpected words just then), 'my dearest heart, my joy, you must realize that everyone is really responsible for everyone and everything.'

> *From*: Dostoyevsky's *The Brothers Karamazov*

I think that we have a moral duty to the family to ensure that an untreated baby survives for as short a time as possible. . . . Over the past year or so we have had a 100% mortality within the first four weeks of life in those infants whom we decided not to treat actively.

*From*: H. Eckstein: 'Spina Bifida, the Surgeon's Responsibility', as cited by Richard Nicholson: 'Should the Patient be Allowed to Die?' *Journal of Medical Ethics* 1975

## 2.1   INTRODUCTION: STATING THE PROBLEM

ONE way of trying to combine the Sanctity-of-Life Principle (SLP) with a limited duty of life-preservation is to argue for the truth of the principle of double effect. According to this principle, a morally relevant difference exists between what one intends and what one merely foresees as a non-intended consequence of one's action or omission. Whilst there are, according to the principle of double effect, some acts wrong in themselves (such as intentionally killing the innocent), it may nevertheless be permissible to allow death to occur as a non-intended side-effect of some other action that is performed for a proportionate reason. For the principle of double effect to be of any moral interest, it must thus rest on the presupposition that one is not, or is at any rate less or differently, responsible for the foreseen but non-intended consequences of an action or an omission. I shall argue against the principle of double effect in Chapter 3. In the present chapter, I am concerned with something that appears to be presupposed by the SLP: the view that a distinction can be drawn in terms of causal responsibility, and hence in moral significance, between killing (which is *always* wrong) and allowing to die (which is *not* always wrong). In other words, I am going to examine whether supporters of the qualified SLP can avoid the charge of inconsistency by distinguishing, in a morally relevant way, between instances of killing and (some) instances of allowing to die.

To distinguish killing from letting die, supporters of the sanctity-of-life view frequently appeal to the distinction between acts and omissions. Initially, there would appear to be good reasons for this—for if killing the innocent (an action) is always wrong, and allowing to die (an omission) is at least sometimes permissible, this would seem to presuppose that a morally relevant difference exists between actions or killings on the one hand, and at least some omissions or refrainings on the other. As Daniel Dinello, whose views I will discuss in Sections 2.3 and 2.4, puts it in his defence of the asymmetry implied by the qualified Sanctity-of-Life Principle: doing something (or causing death) is morally somewhat more reprehensible than knowingly doing nothing.[1] However, while it might initially appear plausible to rest a defence of the qualified SLP on the acts and omissions distinction, such attempts are, as we shall see, ultimately unsuccessful.

Let us begin, then, by focusing on the link between a given event, such as a death, and an agent's moral responsibility for that event. Causation provides that link—for it is a necessary condition of an agent's being responsible for an event that it be the consequence of something that the agent does. When an event like death is thus a consequence of an action, such as stabbing or shooting, this is always by way of the causal connection between the given event and the action, and it is this causal connection which enables us to identify the agent and to hold her responsible for the death in question. In other words, the death is a consequence of what the agent *does*.

But can an agent bring about, or cause, an event only by doing something, or also by doing nothing? Common sense and the law recognize that we are causally, and hence prima facie morally and legally, responsible not only for the consequences of our actions but also for the consequences of at least some of our omissions. This is made clear in the previously cited New South Wales (Australia) Crimes Act, which defines 'murder' as follows:

Murder shall be taken to have been committed where the act of the accused, or *the thing omitted by him to be done, causing the death charged*, was done or omitted with reckless indifference to human life, or with intent to kill or inflict grievous bodily harm upon some person.[2]

For the law, causation is of primary importance. For example, during the trial of Dr William Waddill, Jr., the Orange County (California) Superior Court judge, James K. Turner, told the jury: 'You may not find the defendant guilty of murder unless you are satisfied that the defendant, by act or omission, was the proximate cause of the death of Baby Girl Weaver.[3]

Supporters of the SLP agree that (some) omissions can be causes.

[1] Daniel Dinello: 'On Killing and Letting Die', in Steinbock (ed.): *Killing and Letting Die*, 131
[2] Crimes Act, New South Wales, Australia 1900 (NSW) s. 18(1)(a) (my emphasis).
[3] As cited by O. H. Green: 'Killing and Letting Die', *American Philosophical Quarterly* (1980), 195.

As will be recalled, the Vatican's *Declaration on Euthanasia* defines euthanasia as 'an action or an omission which of itself or by intention causes death'[4] and the qualified SLP prohibits both killings and some instances of allowing a patient to die.

While the notion of an agent causing something by an action is, however, relatively unproblematic, the notion of an agent causing something by an omission, and only by a particular kind of omission, is not.

Hart and Honoré, in their now classical account of *Causation in the Law*, were able to write somewhat optimistically in 1959 that 'it is now thought, at least in England, that there is no special difficulty about omissions',[5] but their optimism was ill-founded. Philosophically and legally, omissions have been the subject of much recent debate, especially in terms of the distinction between positive and negative euthanasia, or between killing and letting die. While some distinction like that between killing and letting die is widely employed in the practice of medicine, it has been found that the basis of the distinction is obscure, elusive and (it has been argued), morally irrelevant.[6] What has made the problem obvious is the development of new medical technologies and our greatly increased ability to sustain the lives of the incurably and terminally ill. Death will often not occur until and unless the agent performs a positive action, such as removing an intravenous drip or turning off a respirator. Is such an action an instance of killing or of letting die?

Another prominent problem that forces a re-examination of the issue is that of children born with severe birth defects. While even very seriously disabled infants can now be kept alive, it is often not possible to correct or ameliorate the underlying physical or mental handicap. Because of this, readily available life-sustaining treatments are frequently not employed, and the infants are being allowed to die. But if, in deciding to forego life-sustaining treatment, physicians are deliberately allowing such infants to die, why, it might be asked, is it thought impermissible to employ positive means to provide a more speedy death and hence shorten suffering? What, one might ask, is the basis for sometimes accepting allowing to die and always rejecting killing?

[4] Sacred Congregation: *Declaration on Euthanasia*, 6.

[5] H. L. A. Hart and A. M. Honoré: *Causation in the Law* (London: Oxford University Press, 1959), 131.

[6] For an excellent collection of articles on the killing/letting die distinction, see Steinbock (ed.): *Killing and Letting Die*.

The natural response to this question is that killing involves the physician in *doing* something that brings about death, whereas allowing to die or refraining from preventing death does not. This natural response is, however, flatly contradicted when, in turning off an artificial respirator (an action usually thought to be an instance of allowing to die), the doctor does, in fact, do something that brings about death. Thus, what seems to be the pre-reflective basis of the distinction between killing and allowing to die is simply untenable, and those supporting it and regarding it as morally relevant are challenged either to find an alternative basis for the distinction, or to accept that active withdrawal of life-support is an instance of killing.

Later on in this chapter, I shall argue that the distinction between killing and letting die does not lie in the difference between the doctor 'doing something' to cause death and 'doing nothing' to prevent death, but rather in the causal role of the agent in relation to the death in question. To put the matter thus is, however, not to provide an easy solution to the conceptual and ethical questions. Take the question of omissions: if it is agreed that *some* omissions are, in terms of causal efficacy and moral significance, the equivalent of positive actions, how do we distinguish those occasions when they are from those when they are not?

In *An Introduction to the Principles of Morals and Legislation*, Jeremy Bentham distinguishes between actions and omissions in terms of positive and negative acts: 'By positive are meant such as consist in motion or exertion; by negative such as consist in keeping at rest . . . Thus, to strike is a positive act: not to strike on a certain occasion a negative one.'[7]

However, Bentham does not tell us what this 'certain occasion' is—that is, when a failure to strike is a negative act and when it is not. If a mother does not feed her baby, the baby will die and her failure to feed it will be cited as the cause of the infant's death. On the other hand, if the woman does not feed a stray cat which is dying from want of nourishment, is her not feeding the cat also a cause of the cat's death? To relate this to our present concern: Bentham's account is not very helpful in telling us when a physician's not doing something that would have prevented death is a negative act and when—as a defender of the qualified SLP might want to claim—it is not; when it is merely an instance of doing nothing to prolong life.

---

[7] Jeremy Bentham: *An Introduction to the Principles of Morals and Legislation* (New York: Hafner Publishing Co., 1948), 72.

Some writers—to be discussed in subsequent sections—take the view that omissions have causal status only when our failure to act is a deviation from the normal course of events; others that the ascription of responsibility for omissions must be linked to the role a moral agent has adopted for herself, or to an agent's duties and voluntary obligations. According to these views, we are causally responsible for the consequences of some of our omissions but not for others. But these conceptions of the causal status of omissions face, as we shall see, some very serious problems.

Difficulties must also be faced with regard to positive actions: if some instances of doing something (e.g. giving a lethal injection) are said to be instances of killing and others (e.g. active withdrawal of life-support) are said to be instances of merely not prolonging life or of letting die, how do we identify those occasions where a physician kills from those where she merely lets die?

Philosophy in general and ethics in particular thrive on uncertainties and ambiguities. Not surprising, then, that there has been a recent spate of literature centring on the distinction between killing and letting die, or positive and negative euthanasia. It has been claimed by some that there is no intrinsic moral difference between killing a patient and allowing a patient to die, whilst others have sought to establish that such an intrinsic moral difference exists. Victories have been claimed on both sides, but those in opposing camps have often failed to see what the other side is getting at. This, I believe, is at least partly due to the fact that arguments have frequently revolved around an inadequate analysis of the distinction between killing and letting die in terms of the distinction between acts and omissions.

It is often assumed that killing and letting die, or positive and negative euthanasia, can be differentiated on the basis that they involve, respectively, 'doing something' to cause death and 'doing nothing' to prevent death. It is also assumed that if the distinction between killing and letting die has moral significance, this is so because killing is always worse than letting die. This is, however, not what the qualified Sanctity-of-Life Principle suggests. The qualified SLP prohibits not only all killings but also some instances of allowing to die. In other words, letting die can—on this view—be as bad as killing. But, and this is of course the point at issue, the qualified SLP also permits *some* lettings die. If the qSLP is thus not to be blatantly inconsistent (in, on the one hand, *prohibiting* all killings and some instances of letting die whilst, on the other, also *permitting* some instances of letting die), it must either hold that some lettings die are not instances of the intentional termination of life (and I shall discuss this defence of the qualified SLP in Ch. 3) and/or, our present concern, it must hold that there is a relevant distinction between prohibited killings and lettings die on the one hand, and some other— permissible—instances of letting die on the other.

When developing the qualified SLP in Chapter 1 of this book, I avoided a blatant inconsistency in the statement of the principle by expressing what it prohibits as 'letting die' and what it permits as 'refraining from preventing death': 'It is absolutely prohibited . . . to kill a patient or . . . to let a patient die . . . ; it is, however, sometimes permissible to refrain from preventing death.'

But it is, of course, fairly obvious that a merely verbal characterization of an action or omission as either 'letting die', 'refraining from preventing death', or indeed 'killing' will not in itself establish the consistency or inconsistency of the qualified SLP, nor be sufficient to indicate a distinction in causal efficacy or moral significance in what the agent does. I shall argue that no such difference exists; but to show this it will be necessary to take a closer look at the notion of causation.

In Section 2.2, I shall begin by discussing a common medical practice: the selective non-treatment of infants born with the medical condition known as spina bifida. Many doctors and others believe that letting die can, at least sometimes, be justified, although they also believe that killing would always be wrong. This raises the question of what distinguishes killing from letting die. I discuss some of the usual interpretations of the killing/letting die distinction in Section 2.3 and show that these are inadequate. In Section 2.4, I develop a more plausible account of the killing/letting die distinction in terms of the causal role of the agent in relation to the death in question. Section 2.5 takes up this question of causation in connection with omissions. I examine Hart and Honoré's account of causal responsibility for omissions and reject it as inadequate. In Section 2.6, I develop what appears to be a more adequate account of the causal status of omissions. On this view, omissions have full causal status; and an agent who refrains from preventing death is causing death, and is responsible for it, just as she would be were she to administer a lethal injection. In Section 2.7, I discuss and dismiss some objections to the view that an agent is just as responsible for the consequences of her refrainings as she is for the consequences of her deliberate and voluntary actions.

## 2.2  SELECTIVE NON-TREATMENT OF INFANTS BORN WITH SPINA BIFIDA

It is well known that many physicians rely heavily on the distinction between acts and omissions, or killing and letting die, or—as it is often put—between positive (or active) and negative (or passive) euthanasia. One physician, arguing for the permissibility of allowing some patients to die, puts it thus:

A physician's approach towards the inevitable ending of life may be either active or passive. Death could occur by actively interceding or by passively discontinuing therapy. In the first instance, one directly causes life to end by an overt act, whereas, by discontinuing therapy, one permits death to occur by omitting an act and permitting nature to take its course.[8]

Here we should note that whilst many physicians speak as if death were inevitable irrespective of whether or not life-prolonging treatment is employed, this is often not the case. In many cases, death becomes inevitable only when the decision has been made not to treat, or not to continue to treat, the patient. This is especially true in the field of neonatology, where many handicapped infants who would have died in earlier times can now be kept alive indefinitely by modern medical technology—although often only at the price of a severely impaired quality of life. But here, as in other areas of medicine, doctors approve in principle, and are willing to practice, negative euthanasia, whereas significantly fewer approve of positive euthanasia. For example, according to a survey of paediatricians in the New Haven (USA) area, ninety-eight per cent of paediatricians approved of letting infants die, whereas only thirty-nine per cent approved of positive euthanasia.[9] A more recent survey by the Monash University Centre for Human Bioethics in Melbourne, Australia, showed similar results. In a survey of nearly two hundred obstetricians and paediatricians in Victoria, all but two agreed that in some circumstances it was proper to decide against using all available

[8] Vincent J. Collins, MD: 'Limits of Medical Responsibility in Prolonging Life', *Journal of the American Medical Association* 206 (1968), 390.

[9] R. S. Duff and A. G. M. Campbell: 'Moral and Ethical Dilemmas: Seven Years into the Debate About Human Ambiguity', *Annals of the American Academy of Political and Social Science* 447 (1980), 26.

means to keep an infant alive; yet only thirty-one per cent of obstetricians and forty per cent of paediatricians were prepared to accept that active euthanasia could ever be justified. In other words, ninety-nine per cent of doctors were ready to allow an infant to die, but of these more than sixty per cent were not ready to kill it.[10]

Surveys such as these are confirmed by reports of actual practices in the field of paediatrics and neonatology, and the selective non-treatment of infants born with spina bifida is perhaps the best-documented example.[11]

Spina bifida is the result of faulty embryological development of the spinal cord and the vertebral column. In serious cases of spina bifida, the infant is born with a meningomyelocele, an exposed sac filled with cerebrospinal fluid that contains the infant's defective spinal cord. The sac is often only partly covered by anything resembling normal skin and may leak fluid. Because of this malformation, the child is usually paralysed below the level of the lesion, generally incontinent, and may suffer from hydrocephalus (or water on the brain), which causes a swelling of the head, often brain damage, and if left untreated, eventual death.

Until 1957 most infants afflicted with spina bifida died relatively young. However, in 1958 a new device—a shunt known as the Holter valve—was developed, whereby cerebrospinal fluid could be drained from the brain to the heart. In some hospitals, it became routine practice to make vigorous efforts to keep every spina bifida infant alive. As a consequence, many babies born with this condition were in fact kept alive, but only with varying and different degrees of deformity or disability. Many were severely handicapped, suffering from gross paralysis, deformities of the legs and spine, and were permanently incontinent. Mental retardation was common.

Responding to the poor outlook of many of these infants, one paediatrician, John Lorber in Sheffield, England, presented a number of criteria to mark off those babies with mild deformities who would respond well to surgical treatment from those with severe deformities who would not.[12] Treatment became selective, and many infants that

---

[10] P. Singer, H. Kuhse, and C. Singer: 'The Treatment of Newborn Infants with Major Handicaps: A Survey of Obstetricians and Paediatricians in Victoria', *The Medical Journal of Australia* 2:6 (1983), 274–9.

[11] For a history of the treatment of spina bifida infants and additional references, see Kuhse and Singer: *Should the Baby Live?*, ch. 3.

[12] See, e.g., John Lorber: 'Early Results of Selective Treatment for Spina Bifida Cystica', *British Medical Journal* 4 (1973), 201–4.

could have been kept alive were allowed to die. As one doctor puts it, 'we have had an "epidemic" of babies saved from spina bifida by vigorous treatment . . . This epidemic is now over because more and more people are now practising selective policies.'[13] The principle of selective treatment has thus found wide acceptance and in Britain, has been endorsed by the Department of Health and Social Security in its publication *Care of the Child with Spina Bifida*.[14]

If children are not treated vigorously, they are provided with food and, if thought necessary, pain-killing drugs and sedatives. Their death is not brought about by positive means, but if for example an infection develops, an infection that could quite easily be cleared up with a course of antibiotics, no antibiotics are given, and the child often dies of the infection. Herbert B. Eckstein, a paediatric surgeon, describes the fate of untreated infants in the following terms:

> It is in my opinion quite impossible to kill off such an untreated baby, but if surgical treatment is withheld, then it is only reasonable to withhold other forms of treatment, such as antibiotics, oxygen and tube feeding . . . In our experience to date all children . . . who were refused surgical treatment have died within a month and if a baby is not to be treated, then the surgeon and nursing staff should do nothing to prolong life.[15]

John Lorder takes a similar stance when he states that 'it is essential that nothing should be done which might prolong the infant's survival'. And he goes on to urge doctors to resist the temptation to operate because 'progressive hydrocephalus is an important cause of early death'.[16]

Both Lorder and Eckstein thus support negative euthanasia and reject positive euthanasia. As John Lorber more recently put it: 'even if it [positive euthanasia] were legal, I would certainly never do it'.[17] On the other hand, an American paediatrician involved in the treatment of infants afflicted with spina bifida emphatically states:

[13] Discussion between Drs Eckstein, Hatcher, and Slater: 'Medical Practice—New Horizons in Medical Ethics: Severely Malformed Children—a Taperecorded Discussion', 2 (1973), 287.

[14] *Care of the Child with Spina Bifida* was issued by the Department of Health and Social Security in London in 1973.

[15] Discussion between Drs Eckstein, Hatcher, and Slater: 'Medical Practice—New Horizons', 284.

[16] John Lorber: 'Ethical Problems in the Management of Myelomeningocele and Hydrocephalus', *Journal of the Royal College of Physicians* 10 (1975), 54–5.

[17] John Lorber: 'Commentary I and reply to John Harris "Ethical Problems in the Management of Some Severely Handicapped Children" ', *Journal of Medical Ethics* 7 (1981), 121.

It is time that society and medicine stopped perpetuating the fiction that withholding treatment is ethically different from terminating life. It is time that society began to discuss mechanisms by which we can alleviate the pain and suffering of those individuals whom we cannot help.[18]

For our present purposes, the important question is not whether all infants born with spina bifida should or should not be treated, but rather whether the physician's causal responsibility varies between the following two modes of responding to a particular infant's condition:

1. administering a lethal injection, thus causing the infant's death;
2. not employing life-sustaining treatment, that is, refraining from prolonging life, thus allowing the infant to die.

While it is frequently assumed that a distinction not only in the causal role of the agent but also in moral responsibility for the infant's death can be drawn between (1) and (2), I shall argue that this view is mistaken, and that a doctor is just as responsible for an infant's death she refrains from preventing as she would be were she to kill the infant by administering a lethal injection.

First, however, it needs to be shown that the usual ways of differentiating between killing and letting die in terms of the distinction between actions and omissions are inadequate.

## 2.3   KILLING AND LETTING DIE

Both those arguing for and those arguing against the moral relevance of the distinction between killing and letting die have frequently understood the distinction to consist in the difference between doing something to cause death and doing nothing to prevent death, or—even more basically—between performing and not performing certain movements. As we have seen in the last section, two of the doctors involved in the treatment of spina bifida children, John Lorber and Herbert Eckstein, regard it as 'quite impossible' to kill infants born with spina bifida, but they regard it as quite acceptable to 'do nothing' to prolong such infants' lives, thus allowing them to die.

[18] John Freeman: 'Is there a Right to Die—Quickly?', *Journal of Pediatrics* 80 (1972), 905.

On the other side, in arguing against the moral relevance of the distinction, Carolyn R. Morillo, for example, writes:

Presuming motive, intention, knowledge and cost to be held constant, the only difference between killing and letting die seems to be the presence or absence of some particular bodily movement. With regard to that I feel inclined to say that for rational, decision-making creatures, the mere presence or absence of such movements is simply *not* morally relevant . . .[19]

Again, Daniel Dinello, who suggests that killing is 'morally somewhat more reprehensible than letting die', analyses the distinction in the following way:

(A)  X killed Y if X caused Y's death by performing movements which affect Y's body such that Y dies as a result of these movements.

(B)  X let Y die if

  (a) there are conditions affecting Y, such that if they are not altered, Y will die.

  (b) X has reason to believe that the performance of certain movements will alter conditions affecting Y, such that Y will not die.

  (c) X is in a position to perform such movements.

  (d) X fails to perform these movements.[20]

In many cases, the distinction between killing and letting die appears to rest on the distinction between performing a movement that causes death and not performing one that prevents death. A doctor kills an incurably ill patient by administering a lethal injection of morphine, and that involves, amongst other things, piercing the patient's skin and pressing down the plunger of the syringe. This case suggests that the doctor who kills a patient does something which brings about the patient's death, and this involves bodily movement. On the other hand, if a doctor does not move to resuscitate a handicapped newborn infant, she lets the infant die. Cases like this suggest that the difference between killing and letting die lies, respectively, in the presence and absence of particular bodily movements.

But it is not in the mere difference between doing something to cause death and not doing anything to prevent death that the distinction between killing and letting die consists. Neither the hospital's receptionist nor the obstetrician might perform any bodily movements to resuscitate the handicapped newborn infant. Yet it is only the latter who lets the infant die by refraining from preventing its death. If we are to compare the moral relevance of the distinction between killing and letting die, we must compare intentional actions with intentional omissions. An intentional omission is a *refraining*: it presupposes that an agent who refrains from preventing death has the *ability* and *opportunity* to perform an action, is *aware* of this, and refrains from performing an action that she *believes* would, if performed, save or prolong the infant's life.[21]

This means that the notion of causal agency connects the doctor, but not the receptionist, with an ethically significant state of affairs. Only the doctor 'lets die' by refraining from preventing death. The receptionist does not. This means that doctors like John Lorber and Herbert Eckstein are not simply 'doing nothing' to prolong life: rather, they refrain from preventing deaths that could be prevented.

If there are thus cases where a person who 'does nothing' to prevent death does not refrain from preventing death and hence does not let die, there are also cases where we should want to say that a person killed because she did not do something that would have prevented death. For example, if I gave you a kitten and you put it in the bottom drawer of your desk and left it there without food until it died, you have killed the kitten. If you were to reply that you only let it die, I would point out to you that putting a kitten in a drawer and not feeding it is one way of killing it. And, again, if killing were thought to consist in the presence of some bodily movement the performance of which results in death, then I would have killed the drowning man whom I tried to save when I let go of him because I could no longer keep him afloat. Similarly in a medical setting: if the distinction between killing and letting die were to consist in the difference between moving and not moving, then a doctor who discontinues life-sustaining treatment (by, for example, removing an intravenous drip) with the result that the patient dies has killed the patient; whereas a doctor who notices that an intravenous drip has worked itself loose but refrains from reattaching it, with the result that the patient dies,

---

[21] See Green: 'Killing and Letting Die', 196–8. My discussion of the killing/letting die distinction in this and subsequent sections has greatly benefitted from Green's account, although in Sect. 2.7 I ultimately reject the author's analysis.

has merely let her die. This is highly implausible, and it is not surprising that those analysing the difference between killing and letting die in terms of a movement criterion have found the distinction problematic.

Whilst it may be thought that recognitions such as these show that no morally relevant difference exists between killing and letting die, I want to suggest that they show that the distinction between killing and letting die has been incorrectly drawn: killing and letting die cannot be distinguished in terms of the presence or absence of bodily movements, nor in terms of 'doing something' to cause death and 'doing nothing' to prevent death. Rather, what distinguishes killing from letting die is a difference in the causal role of the agent in relation to the death in question: whether the agent causes the death positively or negatively by, respectively, initiating a course of events that will lead to death, or by refraining from intervening in a course of events not of the agent's 'making' which will, coupled with the agent's refraining, lead to death.

A striking feature of many of the usual discussions of the killing/ letting die distinction is that they say nothing about the causal character of the actions and omissions under discussion. Jonathan Bennett's analysis of the distinction is a case in point. In his much-discussed article 'Whatever the Consequences',[22] Bennett tries to show that the absolutist position (he calls it the 'conservative' position) on killing and letting die is mistaken. On Bennett's interpretation of the absolutist view, it is always wrong intentionally to kill an innocent person, even though it is sometimes permissible to let an innocent person die. But, Bennett argues, that position cannot be sustained.

Bennett's analysis of the killing/letting die distinction is based on the following observation: when an act is a killing, it typically is one of the relatively few movements open to the agent which would result in the death of the person killed. For example, *A* points a loaded rifle at *B*. Most of the movements that *A* could make would not result in *B*'s death. He could aim and shoot at the street lamp, shoot in the air,

---

[22] Bennett: 'Whatever the Consequences'. He has since developed an alternative account, in terms of positive and negative instrumentality, see 'Morality and Consequences', S. M. McMurrin (ed.): *The Tanner Lectures on Human Values*, ii (Salt Lake City: University of Utah Press and Cambridge University Press, 1981), 47–116.

or in any direction other than *A*'s. And there is, of course, an almost infinite number of movements that *A* could make that would not even involve shooting the gun. Of all these alternative ways of moving, only one, or at most very few, would result in the death of *B*: keeping the gun aimed at *B*, *A* pulls the trigger and *B* dies.

On the other hand, when an act is an instance of letting die, there are relatively few movements the agent could perform which would not result in the death of the person. For example, a life-saver (*A*) sees *B* drown close by. Instead of moving in one of the relatively few ways that would result in *A* saving *B*'s life, *A* could perform an almost infinite number of other movements that would result in *B*'s death: turn over the page of his book, gaze at the sea gulls, sing a song, or recite a prayer.

Interpreting the distinction between killing and letting die in this way, and holding other things equal, we may state Bennett's analysis as follows:

1. *X* killed *Y* if *X* moved and *Y* died, and of all the ways in which *X* could have moved, *relatively few* would satisfy the condition: if *X* had moved like that, *Y* would have died.
2. *X* let *Y* die if *X* moved and *Y* died, and of all the ways in which *X* could have moved, *almost all* would satisfy the condition: if *X* had moved like that, *Y* would have died.

However, Bennett's analysis of the killing/letting die distinction is inadequate, as the following examples show.

Mary and Nancy are both diabetics. They are shipwrecked on an uninhabited island that is visited once a week by a pleasure boat. In an uninhabited hut, they find a bottle of insulin sufficient to keep both of them alive until the scheduled arrival of the next boat. However, Mary, thinking of her five dependent children at home (Nancy has no children), is afraid that the next boat will not arrive in time and that she might die were she to share the insulin with Nancy. Mary takes the insulin (moving in one of the relatively few ways that will allow her to get the insulin) and, according to Bennett's analysis, kills Nancy.

Why does Mary 'kill' Nancy when she takes the insulin? Is it not much more plausible to suggest that Mary does not kill Nancy when she takes the insulin, but that she *lets her die* when she keeps it (one of a relatively large number of movements), rather than give it to Nancy?

But, again, is it true that in keeping the insulin, Mary 'lets Nancy die', rather than kills her? Not according to this extended example: after having taken the insulin and kept it for a while, Mary notices that Nancy, who is stronger, is planning to take the insulin away from her. Fortunately for Mary, though, Nancy is afraid of heights. Mary knows that and climbs onto the island's highest rock. Thus, moving in one of the relatively few ways that enable her to keep the insulin, Mary *kills* (?) Nancy. No, in continuing to refrain from giving the insulin to Nancy, Mary lets Nancy die by refraining from preventing her death. Nancy dies of diabetes, a condition not of Mary's 'making'.

If there are thus some instances of letting die, where Bennett's number-of-movement criterion will give the intuitively wrong result (or be ambiguous), there are also some cases where what might, on Bennett's account, appear to be instances of letting die are more properly described as what I want to call instances of 'killing by letting die'.

Here the case of the kitten in the drawer may serve as an example. Do you kill the kitten when putting it in your drawer (one of the relatively few movements that will result in the kitten's death), or do you let it die when instead of feeding it you go on a holiday (one of a relatively large number of movements open to you)? I suggest that you let the kitten die by refraining from preventing its death; but this refraining is, in terms of causal agency, also a killing—had you not put the kitten in the drawer, thus initiating a course of events that is under the circumstances and coupled with your subsequent refraining from feeding the kitten sufficient to bring about the kitten's death, the kitten would not have died. At the same time, your putting the kitten in the drawer is not simply a killing—had you merely put the kitten in the drawer and not also refrained from feeding it, the kitten would not have died; there would have been no death and hence no killing. This means that both your initial positive action (putting the kitten in the drawer) and your subsequent refraining (not feeding it) are, under the circumstances, causally necessary conditions for the kitten's subsequent death. Its death is the consequence of a 'killing' that also involves 'letting die'.

There are thus cases of killing that also involve letting die.[23] It would, however, be naïve to assume that the issue of whether Nancy's or the kitten's death is a consequence of a killing or a letting die can be settled either by relying on our linguistic intuitions or on the basis of the presence or absence of bodily movements. Neither Bennett's account of the distinction between killing and letting die, nor Dinello's above two-dimensional analysis, can adequately take account of these complexities. What is required is an analysis of the distinction between killing and letting die in terms of a tripartite distinction in causal agency.

## 2.4   CAUSAL AGENCY

As we saw in the previous section, Dinello takes the distinction between killing and letting die to involve the difference between *doing something* to cause death and *failing to do something* that would prevent death.[24] This is correct for many instances of letting die where

1. an agent $X$ is not responsible for initiating a course of events that will, coupled with her refraining, lead to $Y$'s death, and
2. where refraining from preventing death consists, as it often does, in not performing an action.

However, whilst Dinello's analysis of the killing/letting die distinction is correct for most cases of killing and letting die (e.g. the doctor giving a lethal injection = killing, versus the doctor refraining from resuscitating the defective newborn = letting die), it does not capture the fundamental basis of the distinction, which lies not in the presence

---

[23] Bennett acknowledges that some instances of killing on his number-of-movement criterion may, in fact, be cases of letting die; and cases of letting die instances of killing. He believes, however, that whether this is so depends, in cases of killings that are also cases of lettings die, on the agent's expectations and the inevitability of the death in question (ibid., pp. 216–17); and in cases of lettings die that are also killings, on 'malice and wanton indifference' (pp. 225–6). This would, however, not help us to categorize the Mary/Nancy case, where the fact that Mary would have expected the death of Nancy and probably regarded it as inevitable would lend weight to the killing side, while the fact that neither malice nor wanton indifference may have been involved would lend weight to the letting die side. Bennett's *overall* theory will thus not help us in cases where we are unsure as to which description—killing or letting die—is appropriate.

[24] Dinello: 'On Killing and Letting Die', 128–31.

or absence of bodily movements but in the causal role of the agent in relation to the death in question.

Take again the previous example of the kitten. You put the kitten in the bottom drawer of your desk, leave it there without food and it dies. We might be inclined to call the kitten's death the result of a letting die because you, unlike the doctor who administers a lethal injection, are not 'directly' doing anything to the kitten that will result in its death. But is it true that you merely let it die? It seems not. For in having put the kitten in the drawer, you have initiated a course of events that will, if you continue to refrain from feeding it, result in the kitten's death. Your action of putting the kitten in the drawer and of keeping it there without food, prevents, as it were, the prevention of the kitten's death.[25] You are thus not merely letting the kitten die because of circumstances not of your making, but the kitten's death is the result of what you have done: it is a killing.

Let me explain why this must be so. One characteristic of a killing is that an agent initiates a course of events that will, under the circumstances, result in the death in question. To initiate such a course of events and to let death eventuate is a killing, regardless of whether the consequent death follows the action in close temporal proximity (e.g. $X$ shooting $Y$ in the heart), or whether it takes time for the consequence to eventuate (e.g. $X$ starving $Y$ to death). Furthermore, to initiate such a course of events is a killing regardless of whether it is intentional, unintentional, justifiable, unjustifiable, blameworthy, and so on. Suppose that Anton gives Bertha a glass of poisoned wine, and Bertha dies as a result. In this case, it is clear that Anton killed Bertha. Now take a second case: Charles gives Diana a glass of poisoned wine that will result in Diana's death in three hours' time. However, after having administered the poison, Charles is conscience-stricken and prepares an antidote. He is ready to give it to Diana but then changes his mind; instead of giving it to Diana, he tips it down the sink. In having an antidote but refraining from giving it to Diana, Charles lets Diana die. But this is not merely an instance of letting die: it is, coupled with Charles's administering the poison, an instance of killing which also involves letting die. Charles refrains from intervening in a course of events, initiated by him, and in thus

---

[25] See also R. I. Sikora: 'Killing and Letting Die: Twelve Cases' (unpublished paper), 3–5. Sikora employs the term 'preventing the prevention of death' to describe some cases that are, in my terminology, instances of lettings die that are also killings.

refraining from preventing Diana's death, allows her to die as a causal consequence of his initial action.[26]

In all essential respects this case is similar to the kitten in the drawer. If you had not put the kitten in the drawer, the kitten would not have died—assuming here as in all other cases under discussion that death would not have occurred from some other cause. The fact that your not feeding it may have been unintentional will not alter the fact that you killed the kitten by starving it to death. You did not refrain from preventing the kitten's death (because you lacked the relevant awareness), but you killed it—albeit unintentionally—when you let it die for want of nourishment.

Here it is important to note that whilst both killing and letting die can be unintentional, an agent cannot unintentionally refrain from preventing death: when shooting at a bill board, you can unintentionally kill the person sitting behind it; you can kill the kitten when you unintentionally let it die for want of nourishment; you can unintentionally let your ageing mother die when, because you forgot to open her letter, you do not bring her the medicine she requires to stave off death; but you cannot unintentionally refrain from preventing death. When refraining from preventing death, the agent must always have the ability and opportunity to perform the action and be aware of this and of the fact that the action, if performed, would avert the death in question. If this were not the case, the phrase 'refraining from preventing death' would be entirely gratuitous.

We are primarily interested in the intentional doings of agents. For the purposes of our discussion I shall therefore assume that an agent who kills or an agent who lets die does so knowingly and deliberately, rather than inadvertently or unitentionally. In other words, when speaking about 'letting die', 'not prolonging life', and so on, I shall assume—unless otherwise indicated—that the agent who lets die is *refraining* from preventing death.

What we need to note next is that refraining from preventing death

---

[26] In all these cases the problems raised by Judith Jarvis Thomson in 'The Time of a Killing', *Journal of Philosophy* (1971), 115–32, are obvious. If Jones shoots Smith at $t^1$ and if, as a result, Smith dies at $t^2$, when did Jones kill Smith? Thomson shows that cogent objections can be raised against any of the obvious answers. The problem is not made any easier if not only killing but also refraining from preventing death is involved. When did Charles bring about Diana's death? I have no solution to the problem but will, for the purposes of this chapter, treat 'killing' and 'refraining from preventing death' as conditions necessary under the circumstances for the occurrence of the death in question, leaving moot the issue as to when the bringing about of death occurred. See also n. 70.

need not consist in an agent failing to do something that would, if done, prevent death. An agent can refrain from preventing death by *doing* something—for example, turning off an artificial respirator, removing an intravenous drip, telling the nurse not to administer antibiotics, and so on. Similarly in a non-medical setting: I can refrain from preventing the drowning swimmer's death by removing my hand that held her head above water. If I neither pushed the drowning woman in, nor in any other way positively contributed to her being in the water, I have not killed her if she drowns following the removal of my hand: I let her die. The same applies in the medical setting: if a physician turns off an artificial respirator sustaining the victim of an accident, who is unable to breathe by herself, she has not killed the patient but let her die. In turning off the respirator, the physician refrains from continuing to prevent the patient's death and allows the patient's death to occur as a causal consequence of a medical condition not of her making. The patient would have died earlier from the medical condition, for which the doctor is not causally responsible, had the doctor not intervened and temporarily halted the flow of events that would, without her intervention, have led to the patient's earlier death. It is true that the patient would not have died when she did had the doctor not turned off the respirator, but it is equally true that the doctor's refraining could only result in the patient's death because of, and in conjunction with, the patient's medical condition. Whilst turning off an artificial respirator thus involves the physician in *doing something*, it is essentially different from an act of killing, such as giving a lethal injection. When the doctor administers a lethal injection, she initiates a course of events that is, under the circumstances, sufficient to bring about death.

This means that there are killings that do not require *immediate* physical movements, as—for example—when you sit motionless at your desk, letting the kitten die for lack of nourishment; or when a company, manufacturing a potentially lethal substance, such as asbestos (thought to be relatively harmless until recently), does not advise its customers of ten years ago of the substance's potentially lethal effects; and there are cases of letting die where immediate physical movement is involved: my removing my hand from under the chin of the drowning woman, and the doctor turning off the artificial respirator.

It is thus not 'doing something' versus 'doing nothing' that distinguishes killing from letting die, but rather the difference between an agent initiating a course of events that will lead to death and an agent refraining from intervening in a course of events, not initiated by her, that will also lead to death.

This account can be schematized in the following way:

(A) *X kills Y if*
    (a) there is a causal process $c$ that will lead to $Y$'s death
    (b) $X$ initiates $c$ with respect to $Y$
    (c) $Y$ dies as a consequence of $c$.

(B) *X kills Y if she refrains from preventing Y's death if*
    (a) there is a causal process $c$ that will lead to $Y$'s death unless $X$ or some other agent intervenes and does something $s$ that will stop the process $c$ before $Y$'s death occurs
    (b) $X$ has initiated $c$ with respect to $Y$
    (c) $X$ refrains from doing $s$
    (d) $Y$ dies as a consequence of $c$.

(C) *X lets Y die if she refrains from preventing Y's death if*
    (a) there is a causal process $c$ that will lead to $Y$'s death unless $X$ or some other agent intervenes and does something $s$ that will stop process $c$ before $Y$'s death occurs
    (b) $X$ did not initiate $c$
    (c) $X$ refrains from doing $s$
    (d) $Y$ dies as a consequence of $c$.[27]

The above account makes it clear that any absolutist principle which prohibits the intentional causation of death must, if it is to be consistent, not only prohibit (A) but also (B). In both cases, (A) and (B), an agent $X$ is causally responsible for initiating a course of events that will—either with or without $X$'s subsequent refraining—lead to $Y$'s death. In other words, positive causal agency connects the concepts in such a way that they must necessarily fall under the same moral scheme. Whilst this conclusion may strike many as so self-evidently obvious that it hardly needs explication, it is not without moral bite. If it could be shown, for example, that the policies of leading capitalist countries are causally responsible for the depressed economies, and hence for starvation and death from easily preventable disease in third world countries, then those responsible for the policies would be morally responsible for the deaths of all those

[27] See n. 26 above and also n. 70. (I derived the above scheme from Green: 'Killing and Letting Die', 196–8.)

whose lives they refrain from saving after having initiated a course of events that will, unless someone intervenes, result in their deaths. Whilst much more argument would be required to substantiate this case, this is not my present concern.

Suffice it to note that the absolutist Sanctity-of-Life Principle, to be consistent, would have to prohibit both instances of intentional killings (*A*) and instances of intentional lettings die that are also killings (*B*), because in both cases an agent initiates a causal process which will, either directly or coupled with the agent's refraining, result in a person's death. If we thus understand the SLP as prohibiting actions or omissions that cause death, then we can make some sense of the qualified SLP: whilst it is always wrong for an agent to cause death, it is not always wrong for an agent to refrain from preventing death. In merely refraining from preventing death (*C*), it may be thought, an agent does not *cause* death, but merely allows death to occur as a consequence of a causal process not of her making. I take it, then, that any principle which prohibits actions or omissions which cause death (and that yet allows that an agent may refrain from preventing death), must hold that (*C*) in the above analysis of causal agency is not a case of an agent *X* being causally responsible for *Y*'s death.

This interpretation of the qualified SLP finds support in the Vatican's *Declaration on Euthanasia*,[28] and in the previously cited statement of Judge James K. Turner.[29] It is also consistent with the view of the Protestant theologian, Paul Ramsey, who holds that 'In omission no human agent causes the patient's death, directly or indirectly. He dies his own death from causes that it is no longer merciful or reasonable to fight by possible medical intervention.'[30]

The recognition that, to be consistent, it is not the allowing of death to occur that the SLP prohibits, but rather that an agent be causally responsible for it, has implications for the debate between consequentialism and absolutism.

Let us return to Jonathan Bennett's account of the distinction between killing and letting die, by way of which he wants to show that absolutism is a morally untenable position. Bennett bases his attack on the following obstetrical case: 'A woman in labour will certainly

---

[28] Sacred Congregation: *Declaration on Euthanasia*, 6, 9–11.
[29] See n. 3.
[30] Paul Ramsey: *The Patient as Person* (New Haven: Yale University Press), 1970, 151.

die unless an operation is performed in which the head of her unborn child is crushed or dissected; while if it is not performed the child can be delivered alive, by post-mortem Caesarian section.'[31]

Operating would be killing the child, not operating would be letting the women die. Hence, Bennett suggests, the conservative would choose letting the woman die because killing the innocent is always prohibited. Whilst the non-performance of the operation would also involve the death of an innocent—the mother—the situation is asymmetrical for the conservative 'because the two alternatives involve deaths in different ways: in one case the death is part of a killing, in the other there is no killing and a death occurs only as a consequence of what is done'.[32]

On the assumption that absolutists do not subscribe to the principle 'It is always wrong to kill the innocent, whatever the consequences of not doing so' simply out of blind obedience to a moral authority, they must, according to Bennett, think that the premiss, 'In this case, operating would be killing an innocent human being while not operating would involve the death of an innocent human being only as a consequence of what is done', gives *some* reason for the conclusion 'In this case operating would be wrong'.[33] Bennett's conclusion is that it gives no reason whatever, because it ultimately depends on a morally irrelevant number-of-movement criterion and, he holds, 'I do not see how anyone doing his own moral thinking could find the least shred of moral significance in *this* difference between operating and non-operating.'[34]

However, an absolutist (and not only an absolutist) might, on the basis of considerations of causal agency, reject Bennett's analysis. She might hold that the distinction between killing and letting die in this case lies not in the morally irrelevant number-of-movements criterion, but rather in the difference between an agent being and not being causally responsible for a death. Bennett's analysis, the absolutist might say, is mistaken because it fails to distinguish adequately between an agent doing something that has as a causal consequence a death, and an agent doing something else that does not. In merely refraining from preventing the woman's death, the absolutist might argue, the woman's death is not a consequence of

[31] Bennett: 'Whatever the Consequences', 211.
[32] Ibid., 214.
[33] Ibid.
[34] Ibid., 228.

what the doctor does (e.g. drinking a cup of coffee, sleeping). Rather, the woman's death is a causal consequence of a natural process which the doctor has not initiated and for which she is hence not causally responsible. On the other hand, were she to operate, she would be responsible for the infant's death because she would be initiating a course of events that would lead to death, and this would make her causally responsible for the death. Since we are responsible for what we cause and not for what we fail to prevent (unless there is a special duty to act—and there is no duty to take one life to save another), in not operating, the doctor is not causally responsible for the woman's death: she merely refrains from preventing it.[35] And, the absolutist might conclude her argument, it is in this, the difference in causal agency, that the moral relevance of the distinction between killing and letting die is grounded.

The absolutist's case thus need not rest on the morally irrelevant number-of-movements criterion, and it follows that Bennett's analysis is inadequate to serve as a refutation of absolutism, or of the claim that a morally relevant difference exists between killing and letting die. Rather, what needs to be shown if absolutism is to be refuted (and here, in arguing against the SLP, I very much side with Bennett), is that there is—other things being equal—no difference, either in causal efficacy or in moral significance, between intentionally initiating a course of events that will lead to death and refraining from intervening in a course of events, not initiated by the agent, that will also lead to death: or between instances of (*A*), (*B*), and (*C*) in the above account of causal agency. It is to the showing of this that we must now turn.

## 2.5   CAUSATION AND NORMAL FUNCTIONING

That omissions can have consequences is most poignantly seen when an action omitted to be done is one which is normally expected to be done. Indeed, it is in circumstances such as these that we do quite unhesitatingly attribute the cause of the consequence to the action omitted. If a mother does not feed her infant and the infant dies, then we say that the mother's omission is the cause of the infant's death. Similarly, if a doctor refrains from giving insulin to an otherwise

---

[35] For a defence of such a view see, for example, Elazar Weinryb: 'Omissions and Responsibility', *The Philosophical Quarterly* 30 (1980), 1–18. I shall refer to Weinryb's view in Sect. 2.6.

healthy diabetic patient and the patient dies, then we say that the doctor's omission was the cause of the patient's death. We have certain expectations as to normal functioning, or the normal course of events, and if an agent deviates from them, then we cite her omission, or her failure to do what is expected, as the cause of a consequence, such as death.

Based on the notion of normal functioning, or the normal course of events, Hart and Honoré emphasize that not only actions but also negative events, static conditions, and omissions can be causes:

There is no convenient substitute for statements that the lack of rain was the cause of the failure of the corn crop, the icy condition on the road was the cause of the accident, the failure of the signalman to pull the lever was the cause of the train smash.[36]

The question is, though, whether omissions become causes only when they are deviations from the expected norm. Hart and Honoré think they do. Their account of the causal status of omissions relies heavily on some idea of normalcy:

When things go wrong and we then ask for the cause, we ask this on the assumption that the environment persists unchanged, and something 'has made the difference' between what normally happens in it and what happens on this occasion.[37]

On Hart and Honoré's view, then, the distinction between a 'cause' and a 'condition' can be found in the difference between normal and abnormal functioning:

. . . what is taken as normal for the purpose of the distinction between cause and mere conditions is very often an artefact of human habit, custom or convention. This is so because men have discovered that nature is not only sometimes harmful *if* we intervene, but it is also sometimes harmful *unless* we intervene, and have developed customary techniques, procedures and routines to counteract such harm. These have become a second 'nature' and so a second 'norm'. The effect of drought is regularly neutralized by governmental precautions in conserving water or food; disease is neutralized by inoculation; rain by the use of umbrellas. When such man-made conditions are established, deviations will be regarded as exceptional and so rank as the cause of harm. It is obvious that in such cases what is selected as the cause from the total set of conditions will often be an omission which

[36] Hart and Honoré: *Causation in the Law*, 28–9.
[37] Ibid., 34.

coincides with what is reprehensible by established standards of behaviour . . .[38]

In other words, on Hart and Honoré's account, omissions become
causes when what is omitted to be done deviates from normal
expectations, normal functioning, or normal conditions. However,
whilst the authors are undoubtedly correct in saying that under such
abnormal circumstances we are inclined to become aware of the
causal consequences of omissions, this does not show that omissions
become causes only when they strike us as such, when the act omitted
to be done has become a second nature or a second norm. In making
causation dependent on what happens to be the social norm or
customary practice at the time, Hart and Honoré have, as it were, put
the cart before the horse: in the case of actions, causal responsibility is
a ground for ascribing moral or legal responsibility; in the case of
omissions, however, the order has been reversed. In making causal
connection depend on established practice or normative judgement,
Hart and Honoré cannot, without circularity, ascribe moral responsibility on the basis of causal responsibility. Furthermore, in making
causation dependent on social practice, causation itself has been
relativized. Surely, however, what operates causally in the world to
produce certain consequences does not depend on what happens to
be social practice or normative judgement at the time. Rather, as the
philosopher J. L. Mackie seems to agree in his seminal book on
causation, 'causation . . . is not merely . . . *to us*, but also *in fact*, the
cement of the universe'.[39]

Take the example of selective non-treatment of infants born with
spina bifida discussed in Section 2.2 above. In 1958, after the
development of the Holter valve, it became common practice for a
few years to administer active treatment to virtually all infants born
with this defect, and many infants survived that would have died had
they not received such vigorous treatment. Let us assume that Doctor
*A* thought already then that active treatment was not in the best
interests of all infants because, while it could ensure their survival, it
could not ensure a reasonable quality of life. She adopted certain
selection criteria. A few years later these selection criteria were
accepted by the medical community and it became standard practice

[38] Ibid., 35.
[39] J. L. Mackie: *The Cement of the Universe* (London: Oxford University Press,
1974), 2.

to treat some infants vigorously and to withhold life-prolonging treatment from others. Based on a criterion of normalcy, this would mean that Doctor *A* was causing death in the years following the development of the Holter valve but is not causing death now because selective non-treatment has become the norm. This is odd because, surely, the causal connection recognized in the 1960s between a doctor's failure to treat and an infant's consequent death is still the same today: a doctor omits treatment, and as a foreseen and perhaps desired consequence the infant dies. This example shows that causation cannot depend on what is normal functioning or standard practice.

As I shall argue below, a doctor is causally and prima facie morally responsible for a patient's death—not because doctors normally do prolong the lives of most patients, but because in refraining from preventing death, the doctor's omission is the morally significant cause of the patient's death. If I let an insect be flushed down the sink and it dies, then I am causally responsible for its death—not because it is standard practice not to let insects be flushed down the sink (there are no such norms or expectations), but because I refrained from preventing its death when I could have.[40]

To base causal connection on the notion of normal functioning or customary practice can lead to such implausible antics as those proposed by some legal writers who have taken the analysis provided by Hart and Honoré to its logical conclusion: if causes are but deviations from the norm, might it not follow that not only omissions but also actions are related to their consequences, if any, by way of the notion of normal functioning or normative judgement, rather than normative judgement being based on causal connection? At least one writer takes this view. For J. G. Strand, the overlapping distinctions between normal and abnormal functioning and causing

---

[40] As some of those opposing the 'causation thesis' (i.e. the view that death can be caused by omissions) will be quick to point out, the position developed here has the counter-intuitive result that any absence of an action (or event) is a cause of outcome *Y* if that action or event would have prevented *Y*. This poses the problem, it is sometimes argued, of picking out 'the' cause of anything out of an infinite number of causally necessary conditions; see, e.g., Eric Mack: 'Bad Samaritanism and the Causation of Harm', *Philosophy and Public Affairs* 9 (1980) 230–59, and the reply by John Harris: 'Bad Samaritans Cause Harm', *The Philosophical Quarterly* 32 (1982), 60–9. I shall briefly return to this at the end of Sect. 2.6. Suffice it here to note that this is a general problem about causation and not one of negative causation alone. See also J. L. Mackie: 'Causes and Conditions', in Ernest Sosa (ed.): *Causation and Conditionals* (London: Oxford University Press, 1975), 23 ff.

and permitting become the test for the determination of causal responsibility:

> Under this test, injecting air into a patient's veins could still constitute an act and would be euthanasia, as would be withholding of insulin shots, which do not merely prolong life but whose absence would cause death. However, turning off a life-support system would constitute an omission.[41]

In this quotation, causation has been completely relativized: the causal status of both acts and omissions has been made dependent on what doctors normally do. However, merely to state these cases is to show how unsound it is, philosophically speaking, to base causal responsibility on normal functioning or standard practice.

Similar objections apply to the positions developed by a number of other philosophers. Eric D'Arcy, for example, makes causal responsibility dependent on standard practice and expectations. John Casey maintains that 'If a man does not do $X$, we cannot properly say that $X$ is the cause of some result $Y$ unless, in the normal course of events, he could have been expected to do $X$.' Similarly, P. J. Fitzgerald agrees with Hart and Honoré that causes are deviations from a 'routine procedure'. I have decided not to discuss these writers, for it is obvious that a critique of their positions would be substantially similar to the one I have provided of Hart and Honoré's account.[42]

In the light of the inadequacies of accounts that rely on the idea of normalcy, standard practice, or expectations to establish causal responsibility for omissions, let us take a closer look at the notion of causation.

## 2.6   OMISSIONS AS CAUSES

It is sometimes held that irrespective of any other possible deficiencies, analyses of causal responsibility such as that provided by Hart and Honoré[43] are defective because they are based on the quasi-legal fiction that omissions have causal consequences, which they do not.

---

[41] J. G. Strand: 'The "Living Will": The Right to Death with Dignity', *Western Reserve Law Review* 26 (1976), 485. See also George P. Fletcher: 'Prolonging Life: Some Legal Considerations', in Steinbock (ed.): *Killing and Letting Die*, 53.

[42] Eric D'Arcy: *Human Acts* (Oxford: Clarendon Press, 1963); John Casey: 'Actions and Consequences', in John Casey (ed.): *Morality and Moral Reasoning* (London: Methuen, 1971), 180; P. J. Fitzgerald: 'Acting and Refraining', *Analysis* 27 (1973, 133–9). For a critique of some of the above positions, see John Harris: *Violence and Responsibility* (London: Routledge and Kegan Paul, 1980), 30–42.

[43] Hart and Honoré: *Causation in the Law*.

Elazar Weinryb, for example, argues that 'omissions have no consequences, since they lack causal efficacy', and from this he draws the conclusion that we have, in the absence of other duties or voluntary obligations, 'no ground for holding [the Bad Samaritan] responsible for the death of [a] drowning man' whom he could quite easily have saved.[44] Similarly, in the previously cited passage, Paul Ramsey holds that 'in omission no human agent causes death'.[45] And, again, Robert Veatch argues that 'only if physicians caring for dying patients have a specific obligation to provide life-prolonging treatment would they be responsible for an omission'.[46]

Views such as the above also underlie the distinction many practising physicians draw between killing a patient and letting a patient die. As one previously cited doctor, Vincent J. Collins, puts it: 'When one permits death by not continuing therapy, the harm that is done is done by nature acting . . .'.[47]

In this section, I shall be concerned with two interrelated tasks: in demonstrating just how it is that omissions can be causes and hence have consequences, I shall not only show that those who deny causal efficacy to omissions are mistaken, but shall at the same time provide an account of causal responsibility that avoids the deficiencies previously identified in Hart and Honoré's and similar analyses.

As we saw in the previous section, social norms and expectations may explain why we see one factor as more important or more significant than another in causally contributing to a consequence, but social norms or expectations cannot provide an adequate characterization of what it is to be a cause. To determine the latter, it will be necessary to go beyond the relativity imposed by the notion of 'normalcy' and to examine causation as a feature, or cluster of features, that operates in the world independently of what happens to be customary practice or social norm.

David Hume provided not one but two definitions of causation. He wrote:

We may define a cause to be *an object followed by another, and where all the objects, similar to the first, are followed by objects similar to the second*. Or, in

[44] Weinryb: 'Omissions and Responsibility', 3, 17.

[45] Ramsey: *The Patient as Person*, 151.

[46] Robert M. Veatch: *Death, Dying, and the Biological Revolution* (New Haven: Yale University Press, 1976), 92.

[47] Collins: 'Limits of Medical Responsibility', 390; see also n. 8.

other words, *where, if the first object had not been, the second never had existed.*[48]

While Hume's first definition is linked to present-day regularity analyses, his second definition (which is *not* a restatement of the first) is linked to contemporary counter-factual analyses of causation. The account J. L. Mackie provides of causation accommodates both regularity and counter-factual analyses. I will use it as a basis for a sketch of how it is that omissions can be causes and can be identified as such against the background of a field of causal conditions.[49]

Before embarking on this, a disclaimer is in order: the concept of causation is complex and the literature concerning it vast. A detailed analysis of causation would go far beyond the scope of a book on the sanctity-of-life doctrine in medicine. The account of causation that I am going to provide is hence necessarily limited; it will, however, be sufficient to show that omissions can be causes, and that an agent is, other things being equal, just as responsible for a consequence she refrains from preventing as she is for a consequence she brings about by a deliberate action.

Whilst Hume often speaks as if it were pairs of single events that are causally related to each other, Mill points out that

It is seldom if ever between a consequent and a single antecedent that invariable sequence subsists. It is usually between a consequent and the sum of several antecedents; the concurrence of all of them being requisite to produce, that is, to be certain of being followed by, the consequent.[50]

One of Mill's examples is that of a person dying after having eaten a certain dish. Mill recognizes that we might want to say that the cause of that person's death was the eating of that particular dish. But, Mill points out, the eating of that dish is not sufficient to produce death. The eating of the dish may only have this effect when combined with a 'particular bodily constitution, a particular state of present health, and perhaps even a certain state of the atmosphere'.[51] The cause then is, according to Mill: 'philosophically speaking . . . the sum total of the conditions positive and negative taken together; the whole of the contingencies of every description, which being realized, the consequent invariably follows'.[52]

[48] David Hume: *An Enquiry concerning Human Understanding*, section vii (New York: Collier Books, 1962), 89.

[49] Mackie: *The Cement of the Universe*.

[50] J. S. Mill: *A System of Logic* bk. iii, ch. 5, sect. 3 (London: Longman's, 1959), 214.

[51] Ibid.

[52] Ibid., 217.

Whilst Mill is aware that we may be tempted to call the eating of the dish the cause of death, since this event was 'nearest' to the consequence, it does not follow that the other conditions were any less essential in producing death.[53] Mill thus insists on the *complexity* of causes. He does, however, also insist on their *plurality*: 'Many causes may produce mechanical motion: many causes may produce some kind of sensation: many causes may produce death.'[54]

Plurality and complexity of causes are, however, two quite distinct notions. It is important to keep this in mind because it is easy for lawyers and doctors to confuse the two concepts when inquiring for the cause of death on the basis of a Millian analysis of causation. For example, it is sometimes argued that in cases where life-support is withdrawn or withheld, the disease and not the doctor causes the patient's death. However, whilst death from disease is one cause of death out of a plurality of possible complex causes (by drowning, stabbing, poisoning), it does not follow that the disease is 'the cause' of death in a medical setting where a minimally sufficient condition for death obtains only if the doctor also refrains from treating. This is something to which I shall revert below.

J. L. Mackie, in building on Mill, describes his account of causation as a modification and improvement of the (Humean) view that a cause is a necessary and sufficient condition.[55] Suppose, he says, that a fire has broken out in a certain house, and that experts investigating the cause of the fire conclude that it was caused by an electrical short-circuit at a certain location. What, Mackie asks, is the exact force of their statement that this short-circuit caused this fire? It cannot mean, Mackie holds, that the short-circuit was a necessary condition for this house's catching fire at this time, because there were many other things that could have resulted in the house catching fire: the overturning of a lighted stove, a short-circuit in a different place, and so on. Equally, Mackie suggests, the experts cannot mean that the short-circuit was a sufficient condition for this house catching fire;

---

[53] Donald Davidson takes a different approach, distinguishing causes from their descriptions and treating 'the' cause of a consequence such as death as the *whole* cause; see Donald Davidson: 'Causal Relations', in Myles Brand (ed.): *The Nature of Causation* (Chicago: University of Illinois Press, 1976) 353–67. However, see also Frank Jackson's review of Myles Brand (ed.): *The Nature of Causation, Journal of Symbolic Logic* 42 (June 1982), 470–3.

[54] Mill: *A System of Logic*, bk. iii, ch. 10, 286.

[55] Mackie: 'Causes and Conditions', 15. (The following analysis of Mackie's position was inspired by an unpublished paper of Joy Melgaard and I wish to thank her for initiating my thinking in this direction.)

because if the short-circuit had occurred but there has been no inflammable material nearby, the fire would not have started. But if the electrical short-circuit was neither necessary nor sufficient to cause the fire—in what sense, Mackie asks, can it then be said to have caused the fire?[56]

It can be said to have caused the fire because, Mackie holds, it is an *inus* condition, that is, 'an *insufficient* but *non-redundant* part of an *unnecessary* but *sufficient condition*'.[57] The electrical short-circuit was *insufficient* to produce the fire because some positive and negative conditions (including the presence of inflammable material and the absence of a sprinkler) contributed equally to the fire; however, in *this particular* situation, the short-circuit was also *non-redundant* in producing the fire, because without it the fire would not have started. Together, the short-circuit and the presence of inflammable material, the absence of the sprinkler and so on, constituted a situation that was *sufficient* to produce the result, but that situation was also *unnecessary* in that the fire could have started in some other way.[58]

Mackie formalizes this account in the following way: If '*A*' stands for a 'type of event situation' (for example, the occurrence of the short-circuit), and '*B*' and '*C̄*' stand for other positive and negative conditions (presence of inflammable material, absence of a sprinkler), then the conjunction '*ABC̄*' constitutes what Mackie calls a 'minimal sufficient condition' for the fire.[59] If there is a necessary and sufficient condition for this result, then a collection of disjuncts of similar groups of *inus* conditions comprises what Mackie calls the 'full cause'.[60]

As Mackie puts it:

The formula '*ABC̄* or *DĒF* or *ḠH̄I* or . . .' represents a necessary and sufficient condition for the fire, each of its disjuncts such as '*ABC̄*', represents a minimal sufficient condition, and each conjunct in each minimal sufficient condition, such as '*A*' represents an *inus* condition.[61]

What we select as a cause is an *inus* condition that operates against the background of a causal field, where what happens to be part of the causal field on a particular occasion is, according to Mackie,

[56] Ibid., 15–16.
[57] Mackie: *The Cement of the Universe*, 62.
[58] Ibid.
[59] Idem: 'Causes and Conditions', 17.
[60] Idem: *The Cement of the Universe*, 64.
[61] Idem: 'Causes and Conditions', 17. Each disjunct is thus one of a plurality of possible causes in Mill's sense—see n. 54.

automatically ruled out as being a cause.[62] How the causal field is defined differs according to the particular questions we are concerned with asking.

Mackie illustrates the notion of different causal fields by way of the following example:

> What caused this man's skin cancer may mean 'Why did this man develop skin cancer now when he did not develop it before?' Here the causal field is the career of this man: it is within this that we are seeking a difference between the time when skin cancer developed and times when it did not. But the same question may mean 'Why did this man develop skin cancer, whereas other men who were also exposed to radiation did not?' Here the causal field is the class of men thus exposed to radiation. And what is the cause in relation to one field may not be the cause in relation to another. Exposure to a certain dose of radiation may be the cause in relation to the former field: it cannot be the cause in relation to the latter field since it is part of the description of that field, and being present throughout that field it cannot differentiate one sub-region of it from another. In relation to the latter field, the cause may be . . . 'some as-yet-unidentified constitutional factor'.[63]

It is obvious from this account that a certain arbitrariness is involved in what we pick out as the cause of a consequence, because what is a cause cannot be part of the causal field; and the causal field, Mackie points out, tends to be the normal course of events, whilst what is selected as the cause is a deviation from the norm.[64] This means that what we normally call the cause of an event is not 'the cause' at all (because this is a minimally sufficient condition that operates independently of our expectations), but rather a reflection of 'some conversational or other purpose of the speaker'.[65]

How, then, is this arbitrariness—also recognized by Hart and Honoré—to be avoided? Hart and Honoré, for example, note that 'the cause of a great famine in India may be identified by the Indian peasant as the drought, but the World Food Authority may identify the Indian Government's failure to build up reserves as the cause and the drought as a mere condition'.[66]

As I argued in the preceding section, Hart and Honoré's solution in terms of 'normal functioning' is inadequate because on their account causal responsibility depends on social norms, rather than social

---

[62] Ibid., 22.
[63] Ibid.
[64] Idem: *The Cement of the Universe*, 35.
[65] Ibid., 36.
[66] Hart and Honoré: *Causation in the Law*, 33.

norms on causal responsibility. Mackie's view is an improvement on Hart and Honoré's account: any factor which is an *inus* condition is a cause in the correct sense of the word. However, only certain of these will be worth citing as causes, depending on the questions we are concerned with asking. For moral and legal purposes, Mackie points out, we often want to know what caused a certain event with a view to how it could, and perhaps should, have been prevented.[67]

Take the example of the house on fire. The fact that the house existed was a necessary condition for the fire breaking out, and so a cause of the fire. And this was a cause to the same extent that the presence of inflammable material, the absence of a sprinkler, and the occurrence of a short-circuit was. However, it is not as relevant to cite the existence of the house as a cause; by identifying the short-circuit, the presence of inflammable material or the absence of a sprinkler as a cause, we provide information that is relevant to the prevention of fires; mentioning the house as a cause is not. It is thus in the light of these purposes directed at the prevention of undesirable or harmful consequences that certain causes, that is, *inus* conditions, are more prominent than others.[68]

It is obvious, then, that in the social and ethical context where we are concerned with the avoidance or alleviation of certain harmful consequences, such as death, human actions and omissions will figure prominently as causes of harm. Considerations as to how undesirable consequences can be avoided will make certain actions or omissions more significant than other conditions and thus more relevant to be cited as causes. Here it should be emhasized that it is not their significance which *makes* them causes, but rather this significance makes it relevant to cite them as such. In other words, what becomes a prominent cause will, in the social context, depend on how relevant it is in bringing about or avoiding certain consequences.

It is, however, precisely in the social context that analyses of causation based on social norms and expectations become problematic. What, as John Harris poignantly asks,

if normal functioning is always a disaster? Every year, just like clockwork, the poor and the jobless, the aged and the infirm, suffer terribly and many of them die. What is the cause? The myopic view is that they die because they are

[67] Mackie: *The Cement of the Universe*, 35.

[68] Here we might be inclined to cite the short-circuit as 'the cause' because it is somehow 'closest' to the outbreak of the fire; once again, though, this does not mean that the short-circuit was causally any more 'necessary' or important than the other *inus* conditions.

poor and jobless, aged and infirm. That is what distinguishes them from those
who do not suffer, from those who do not die. But the World Moral
Authority may identify the neglect of other members of society or of the
government as the cause . . . And surely the World Moral Authority's causal
explanation is not upset by the discovery that this society normally neglects
its weakest members, that there is no difference between what they did this
year and what they always do . . .[69]

Similarly, in a medical context: each year thousands of handicapped infants are allowed to die. What is 'the cause'? The 'myopic
view' is that they die because they have pneumonia, or some other
infection that, if left untreated, leads to death. But here again, the
'World Moral Authority's' causal explanation may identify the
deliberate non-treatment as 'the cause' of death, even though there is
no difference between what doctors have done on these particular
occasions and what they always do in the case of severely handicapped infants.

If the cause of death of many infants born with spina bifida was,
prior to the availability of antibiotics, appropriately identified as an
infection, this causal explanation is no longer the appropriate one for
moral purposes. If antibiotics that will prevent death are available,
and if they are deliberately withheld from an infant, then a new *inus*
condition, namely the doctor's omission to employ an available
means to prevent death, must be added as a conjunct to the minimally
sufficient condition that in the past brought about death if an
infection, such as meningitis or pneumonia, occurred. If the question
we are concerned with is how death could or should have been
prevented, then the doctor's failure to employ an available means
that would have prevented death will be the most significant, and
morally relevant, cause of the infant's death.[70]

If we ask, however, how death *could have been prevented*, then we

[69] Harris: *Violence and Responsibility*, 41.

[70] It might be objected that the account of causation developed here is somewhat
implausible because it implies that bringing about the existence of a child (conceiving
it) is to cause its death; similarly, my account of causal agency developed in Section 2.4
would imply that conceiving is killing because it initiates a causal process that will lead
to death. It is true, of course, that conception is, strictly, a cause of death because had
the child not been conceived, 'it' could not have died (just as in Mackie's example, had
the house not existed, 'it' could not have caught fire). Similarly again, giving birth to a
child and then not feeding it: does this mean that giving birth is the cause of death?
However, if we are, for moral and legal purposes, concerned with the prevention of
certain consequences, such as deaths, then we must presuppose the existence of those
whose deaths we are trying to prevent and it will not be relevant to cite conception,
birth, or a person's having a mortal body, as a morally significant cause of death.

are approaching the question of causation in terms of a counter-factual account, where—according to Hume's second definition of causation—'*if the first object had not been, the second never had existed*'.[71]

Mackie's account, it would seem, also sustains counter-factual and other conditional analyses associated with causation.[72] Mackie offers the following example:

If $A\bar{B}\bar{C}$ are the minimally sufficient conditions for a person's death, where $A\bar{B}\bar{C}$, respectively, stand for eating a certain (poisoned) dish, not taking an antidote and not having one's stomach evacuated, and if none of the other minimally sufficient conditions was realized on this occasion (e.g. death by drowning, shooting, stabbing), then it follows that if $\sim A$ then $\sim$(result) $P$, that is, 'if he had not eaten of that dish, he would not have died.[73] It is obvious that such counter-factual analyses are of importance in the medical context, where very often and independently of social expectations, a patient would not have died had the doctor not refrained from administering anti-biotics, refrained from operating on a malformed child, and so on.

Of course, on Mackie's account it would also be true that had the person eaten the dish but also had his stomach evacuated he would not have died (if $C$ then $\sim P$). Similarly, in the medical example: the patient would not have died even if the doctor had refrained from administering antibodies, had she not also suffered from, say, pneumonia. In what sense, then, can we say that the doctor's omission, rather than the pneumonia, is the cause of a patient's death?

To answer this question, we need to return to Mackie's notion of a causal field. As Mackie's example of skin cancer indicates, we can raise questions such as 'What is the cause in death?' in different causal contexts. Take the example of an infant born with spina bifida who develops pneumonia, is not treated with antibiotics, and subsequently dies. What is 'the cause' of the infant's death? If the question is raised within the context of spina bifida children selected for non-treatment, a satisfactory answer would be that the cause of death was pneumonia. Here the causal field is the medical history of an untreated spina bifida infant, and it is within this field that we are seeking to establish what 'made the difference' between the time when

[71] See n. 48.
[72] Mackie: *The Cement of the Universe*, esp. ch. 2 and pp. 64–5.
[73] Ibid., 64.

death occurred and when it did not. In this context, the fact that the infant contracted pneumonia will allow us to differentiate between the time when the infant died and when it did not. However, whilst the selection of such a restricted causal field will undoubtedly be relevant for the answering of certain questions, someone concerned to establish whether all human lives are treated equitably in the practice of medicine might phrase the question in the following way: 'Why do spina bifida children who contract penumonia die, whereas other infants not afflicted with spina bifida who also contract pneumonia do not?' Here the causal field is the class of infants who contract pneumonia in a hospital setting. And, as Mackie points out, the cause of death in relation to one field may not be the cause of death in relation to another. Pneumonia may be the cause of death in relation to the former field, it cannot be the cause in relation to the latter 'since it is part of the description of that field, and being present throughout that field it cannot differentiate one sub-region from another'.[74]

What, then, is the cause of an untreated infant's death if pneumonia is ruled out as a possible cause? If it can be shown that what differentiates those situations in which death occurs (or would have occurred) from other situations in which death does not occur (or would not have occurred) is the doctor's failure to treat, then the doctor's omission is the causal factor that allows us to distinguish those situations in which death occurs from those in which it does not, and the doctor's failure to treat is identified as the causal factor that made, or would have made, the difference between an infant's dying or not dying. Hence, the doctor's failure to treat is the cause of death.[75]

The above account of causation avoids the relativity of Hart and Honoré's analysis, where as we saw, the causal status of omissions depends on the notion of normal functioning and standard practice. Mackie's account of causation breaks the circle of relativity imposed by reliance on the idea of normalcy and shows that omissions have the same causal efficacy as actions in bringing about a consequence,

[74] Mackie: 'Causes and Conditions', 22.

[75] See also my discussion of the trial of the English paediatrician Dr Leonard Arthur for the death of the Down's syndrome infant John Pearson—'A Modern Myth: That Letting Die is not the Intentional Causation of Death: Some Reflections on the Trial and Acquittal of Dr Leonard Arthur', *Journal of Applied Philosophy* 1: (1984) 21–38; also Bart Gruzalski: 'Killing and Letting Die', *Mind* 40 (1981), 91–8, for an account of causal responsibility similar to that developed above.

such as death. Moreover, to the extent that omissions are intentional, that is, are instances of an agent *refraining* from preventing death, the agent is not only causally but also prima facie morally responsible for those consequences. The Bad Samaritan is thus, contrary to Elazar Weinryb, both causally and prima facie morally responsible for the death of a drowning man, whom he could quite easily have saved.[76] Similarly doctors: to refrain from sustaining life, or to let die, is to cause the patient's death, and to be prima facie morally responsible for it, irrespective of whether, as Robert Veatch appears to think necessary, the doctor has a specific obligation to provide life-sustaining treatment.[77]

The point is this: I can refrain from preventing someone's death, regardless of whether or not I have a duty to prevent that person's death; and if I can and do refrain, then I am not only causally but also prima facie morally responsible for the consequences of my omissions. I may well have a duty to prevent someone's death, but it is only when I refrain from preventing it that I infringe the duty. If someone dies without my refraining, then I am—other things being equal—not morally responsible for it, and have not infringed any duty to prevent death. Hence Veatch is mistaken to assume that if I do not have a special obligation to provide life-prolonging treatment, I am not responsible for a death I refrain from preventing. Causal responsibility, coupled with the notion of refraining, is primary—not the existence of particular duties.[78]

Before concluding this section, it is necessary to draw out a distinction that has been implicit all along: the distinction between causal and moral responsibility.

### 2.61   Causal Responsibility

If an agent *A* did not do *X*, where *X* would have prevented *Y*'s death, *A*'s not doing *X* is a cause of *Y*'s death. If, however, *A* merely does nothing to prevent *Y*'s death and does not *refrain* from preventing it, then she will generally not be morally responsible for the death, since she lacked the ability, opportunity, or awareness necessary for her to be able to prevent *Y*'s death.[79]

---

[76] See n. 44.

[77] See n. 46.

[78] See also Green: 'Killing and Letting Die', 202–3.

[79] We should note here, though, that for example the fact that an agent is unaware of the consequences of her doings or refrainings is not always an adequate excuse. Her lack of awareness may be due to negligence.

Here it may be objected that the view that death and other consequences may be caused negatively by omissions (the 'causation thesis') must lead to the implausible general claim about negative causation: that any absence of any action (or event) is a cause of outcome $Y$ if that action or event would have prevented $Y$, whether or not this action or event was possible at all.[80]

What, those opposing the causation thesis might ask, allows us to promote any of the infinite number of causally necessary conditions to the status of a cause, or 'the cause' of anything? Or, to put it another way: what allows us to restrict the number of causes to a manageable group? However, whilst the question of what allows us to identify one of the infinite number of causally necessary conditions as 'the cause' is undoubtedly complex, it was already noted above that this is a general problem about causation, both positive and negative, and not one for negative causation alone.[81] Moreover, Mackie's account of causation, making use of the notions of causal fields and *inus* conditions within particular fields, goes, I believe, a long way towards overcoming some of these very vexing problems.[82]

In addition to this general argument about negative causation, more specific arguments are sometimes offered as to why we should not say that *causally possible* actions or events are the cause of anything. Eric Mack offers such an argument in terms of Jones's failure to save Smith from drowning:

If one concedes that conditions *not* including the absence of rescue actions are jointly sufficient for Smith's drowning when Jones' refraining from rescue activity is not possible, then why believe that the factor which renders this refraining possible also has the effect of rendering the previously jointly sufficient conditions for Smith's drowning insufficient for that harm? To believe that, when Jones' refraining is possible, the absence of rescue activity by Jones is a cause of Smith's drowning, but that otherwise the absence of that action is not a cause of that harm is to be committed to a certain causal proposition. This proposition is that the factor which transforms the situation into one in which refraining is possible (for example, Jones notices the struggling Smith, Jones comes to believe that he can save Smith) has the specific effect of altering the causal sufficiency of that group of conditions previously sufficient for the drowning.[83]

As John Harris notes, Mack is here making use of an argument of

---

[80] For such an objection, see, e.g., Mack: 'Bad Samaritan', 241.
[81] See n. 40.
[82] See Mackie: 'Causes and Conditions', esp. 23–7.
[83] Mack: 'Bad Samaritanism', 255.

Elizabeth Anscombe's concerning 'believable effects'.[84] Mack suggests that it is not believable that the simple fact that an agent changes her beliefs could alter the causal sufficiency of that group of conditions that was previously sufficient to bring about a death. But this is clearly false. Let us assume that prior to the development of antibiotics, all spina bifida infants who contracted a particular infection died. Let us assume next that after the development of antibiotics this type of infection can be cured. A doctor knows this and believes that by using antibiotics she can avert the deaths of those spina bifida infants who contract the infection. Quite clearly, this means that those conditions previously sufficient for death are no longer sufficient now: a new *inus* condition—the agent's refraining from preventing death—must be added to the previously minimally sufficient condition for death (the infant being afflicted with spina bifida, contracting an infection, and so on); and it is only when the agent refrains from preventing death that a minimally sufficient condition for death exists. Natural conditions, such as tide and wind, or disease—even if often daunting in their magnitude—are not causally sufficient *of themselves*. They are sufficient only in conjunction with other positive and negative *inus* conditions, of which an agent's refraining may be one.

What we might say, then, is this: whilst *A*'s failure to perform an action *X*, which would have prevented *Y*, is a cause of *Y* (even if it was causally impossible for *A* to do *Y*), *A* did not *refrain* from doing *X* and so is not causally responsible for *Y*. For example, while my not throwing a shield between President John F. Kennedy and his assassin Lee Harvey Oswald was a cause of Kennedy's death, it was not *my* not throwing the shield that caused Kennedy's death. Since I did not have the ability, opportunity, the relevant beliefs, and so on, to prevent Kennedy's death, I did not *refrain* from preventing it and so *I* am not causally responsible for his death, although my not throwing the shield was a cause of Kennedy's death.

## 2.62 *Moral Responsibility*

If an agent *A refrains* from preventing *Y*'s death, *her* not doing *X* is a cause of *Y*'s death, and *A* is prima facie morally responsible for the death because she cannot claim that she lacked the opportunity,

---

[84] Harris: 'Bad Samaritans Cause Harm', 63–4. (Harris refers to Elizabeth Anscombe's paper: 'A Note on Mr. Bennett', *Analysis* 26 (1966), 208.)

awareness, or ability, to prevent *Y*'s death. Had *A* not refrained, *Y* would not have died, and *A* was aware of this at the time.

In this connection it will be helpful to refer to the distinction drawn by H. L. A. Hart between causal responsibility and 'moral liability responsibility', that is, between being causally responsible for a consequence and being liable, or having to answer, for the consequences of one's actions or omissions.[85] While an agent is generally answerable for a consequence of her conduct because she is causally responsible for it, she is not accountable *simply* because she is causally responsible for it. Accountability or moral responsibility arises from the connection between causal responsibility and the character or extent of an agent's control over her actions. Thus it would seem that it is only when an agent *refrains* from preventing death that she is prima facia fully accountable for it, just as accountable or morally responsible as she would be had she brought it about by a deliberate positive action. Precisely what is to count as 'refraining' is a topic that needs further investigation; but for our purposes it is enough to note that when doctors like John Lorber and Herbert Eckstein allow a baby to die, they have the ability, the opportunity, and the awareness necessary to make them fully accountable for the consequences of their omissions—just as accountable or morally responsible as they would be had they brought about the infants' deaths by a deliberate positive action.

## 2.7  SOME OBJECTIONS

In the final section of this chapter, I shall discuss some common objections to the view that there is no intrinsic moral difference between killing and letting die.

### 2.71  *Responsibility*

O. H. Green agrees that agents are both causally and morally responsible for the consequences of their deliberate omissions but holds that 'in view of the difference in the causal role of the agent which distinguishes killing from letting die, there is an essential connection between the [killing/letting die] distinction and the moral responsibility of an agent.'[86]

[85] H. L. A. Hart: 'Postscript: Responsibility and Retribution', in H. L. A. Hart: *Punishment and Responsibility* (Oxford: Clarendon Press, 1968), 212–30.
[86] Green: 'Killing and Letting Die', 201.

In killing, an agent *A* 'does something which is sufficient to bring about *B*'s death', and if *A* acts intentionally, this makes *A* 'fully responsible for *B*'s death'. In letting die, on the other hand, *A* is, according to Green, less responsible for *B*'s death, because whilst *A*'s refraining is 'necessary . . . for *B* to die' and (whilst *A*'s refraining) does causally contribute to *B*'s death, in cases of letting die, *B* is already in danger of dying from a condition 'not of *A*'s making' which is sufficient to bring about *A*'s death, unless *A* or some other agent intervenes and prevents death. In killing, an agent is thus, according to Green, fully responsible—both causally and morally—for a death, whereas in letting die an agent is—both causally and morally—less responsible for a preventable death.[87]

It is difficult to see, though, how Green can sustain this claim if moral responsibility depends—as Green says it does—on its 'essential connection' with the causal role of the agent.

Causal *efficacy* does not, as we have seen, vary between instances of killing and letting die, because (contrary to Green) killing and letting die cannot be distinguished on the basis that the former is a sufficient condition for death whereas the latter is but a necessary one. Both killing and letting die are *inus* conditions in two different minimally sufficient conditions for death. This means that killing and letting die have the same causal efficacy. If the doctor had not given the lethal injection, the patient would not have died. Similarly in cases of letting die: if the physician had not refrained from preventing death, the patient would not have died. And since refraining from preventing death is not simply a matter of 'doing nothing' but rather a deliberate non-intervention in a course of events that will, coupled with the physician's refraining, result in the patient's death, killing and letting die cannot be distinguished in terms of causal agency either.

That causal agency is not different in cases of killing and letting die can perhaps most clearly be seen when letting die requires a positive action, such as turning off a respirator. This is not an instance of killing, because the physician did not initiate the course of events that will, if treatment is discontinued, lead to the patient's death; but the physician is a causal agent of death just as she would be were she to give a lethal injection.

There is *one* (ontological) difference, though, that remains even if we hold other things, such as intention, motivation, cost to the agent, probability of outcome, and so on, equal: killing and letting die can

[87] Ibid.

be distinguished in terms of the *causal role* of the agent—whether an agent is the *initiator* of a causal process that will lead to a person's death; or whether an agent refrains from intervening in a causal process not initiated by her that will also lead to a person's death. This, it would appear, is the residual basis of the killing/letting die distinction: the distinction between 'making it happen' that death occur and 'letting it happen' that death occur.

But can the mere difference in the causal role of the agent allow us to distinguish in a morally relevant sense between killing and letting die? Green thinks it can, and in support of this view cites the case of Kitty Genovese to distinguish the causal role of the agent who kills from the causal role of the agent who lets die.

Kitty Genovese was stabbed to death in a street while a number of apartment dwellers looked on. Before we look at the causal role of those involved, though, we need to note that in this and similar cases other morally relevant factors—such as motivation, cost to the agent, and so on—might incline us to think that such killings are indeed worse than lettings die. The question Green asks us to consider is, however, not whether killings are sometimes worse than lettings die, but rather whether the *causal role*, and only the causal role, of an agent differs in a morally relevant way between killing and letting die.

Green agrees that under the circumstances, both killing and refraining from preventing death were necessary conditions for the death of Kitty Genovese; but he holds that their causal 'status' can be distinguished counter-factually: 'Had the apartment dwellers been away or unable to prevent death, Kitty Genovese would still have been stabbed to death. On the other hand, had the assailant been elsewhere or unable to carry out his attack, she would not have died.'[88]

It is true that had the apartment dwellers been away, Kitty Genovese would still have died. But in that case, the onlookers would not have *refrained* from preventing her death, they would have been *unable* to do so. The same holds for Green's second case: if the assailant had been elsewhere, then Kitty Genovese's life would not have been endangered, and if nobody's life is endangered, an agent cannot refrain from preventing death (or let die). If we want to assess the moral responsibility of agents in cases of killing and letting die, we must compare a situation where an assailant is potentially able to kill, and an onlooker is potentially able to prevent the killing. Hence the

[88] Ibid., 202.

appropriate counter-factual situation would be: 'Had the killer attempted to kill but the onlookers not refrained from preventing her death, Kitty Genovese would not have died.'[89] What Green's distinction in causal status shows is that someone's life must be endangered by an assailant (a disease, or the like) before someone can refrain from preventing death. What it does not show is that in a situation where an agent is able to prevent a death and refrains from doing so, killing is different from letting die—either in terms of causal efficacy, or in terms of causal agency.

Richard Trammel, too, thinks that the person who initiates a process that will, if nobody intervenes, lead to death, is 'more responsible' for the resultant death than the person who refrains from preventing it. He argues as follows:

In general, if $X$ kills $Y$, then $X$ is responsible for $Y$'s death. But if $X$ fails to save $Y$, then $X$ may or may not be responsible for $X$ being in the situation in which $Y$ needs to be saved. The more directly involved $X$ is for $Y$'s needing to be saved, the more responsible $X$ is for helping to rescue $Y$ . . . Finally, a person is not necessarily responsible for someone else's needing to be saved; but he is responsible for the life of anyone he kills.[90]

However, being responsible for the situation in which a person needs to be saved is one thing; being responsible for a preventable death, regardless of how it was that the person in danger came to be in

---

[89] A defender of the view that the causal role of an agent differs significantly between killing and letting die might try to defend her position in the following way: if a doctor had been absent, unable to prevent a patient's death, or if she had simply never been born, then it would still be true that the patient would have died. Hence, the argument might proceed, the doctor's refraining cannot have the same causal status as the patient's potentially lethal disease. This is true: if the doctor had been *unable* to prevent the patient's death, then the doctor's *refraining* would not have been a cause of death since, in that case, it would not have been possible for the doctor to refrain from preventing the patient's death. If, however, a doctor were present and able to prevent the patient's death, then she could either refrain or not refrain from sustaining the patient's life; and in *that* case, had the doctor not refrained from sustaining the patient's life, the patient would not have died. Hence, a doctor's refraining is an *inus* condition for the patient's death, and hence a morally relevant cause in all those cases where the doctor is able to refrain and does refrain. In cases where an agent is *unable* to prevent death, her inability is, strictly, part of the full cause of the patient's death because had the agent been able to prevent the patient's death and had she not refrained, the patient would not have died. However, the notion of an agent's inability to do what would, if done, prevent death is uninteresting from the moral point of view, where—to the extent that 'ought' implies 'can'—inability is generally a morally adequate excuse.

[90] Richard R. Trammel: 'Saving Life and Taking Life', *The Journal of Philosophy* 72 (1975), 135.

that situation, is another. It is certainly true that we should, in general, concentrate on the source of a potential harm, trying to prevent the starting of a causal process that will, without later intervention, lead to death. We should try to prevent assailants from assailing, and if we can't, hold them responsible for what they did. Similarly, we should try and prevent disease from arising that will later, if death is to be avoided, require medical intervention. But having said this, it seems implausible to suggest that an agent like a doctor is not fully responsible for a death she refrained from preventing, even if it is true that she did not initiate the disease process that will, without her intervention, lead to the patient's death. There is, contrary to Trammel, no necessary connection between non-moral causal responsibility and moral responsibility, as the following example will show.

I take Trammel to be saying that an agent $X$ is *causally* responsible for a state of affairs if she has brought it about that the relevant state of affairs prevails. Furthermore, I take Trammel to be saying that if $X$ is causally responsible for a state of affairs that imperils $Y$'s life, then $X$ is '[morally] more responsible for helping to rescue $Y$'.[91] But this is obviously not the case: if a paraplegic accidentally and non-negligently nudges a small child so that she falls into a shallow creek, she is causally responsible for the child being in the creek. But if both the paraplegic and I stand by and do nothing to save the drowning child, then *I* am morally responsible for the child's death, because only I—not the paraplegic—refrained from preventing the child's death. Since the paraplegic is *unable* to prevent the child's death, she does not refrain from preventing it, and inability is generally an adequate moral excuse.[92] Similarly in cases where disease is involved: if I am unaware that I am a carrier of hepatitis, then I may be causally responsible for $Y$ being infected with hepatitis. But the fact that I am causally responsible for $Y$'s having hepatitis does not mean that were

[91] Ibid. I say 'I take Trammel to be saying' because Trammel's argument is unclear in so far as he does not distinguish between causal and moral responsibility, and appears to be using the term 'responsibility' interchangeably to stand for either or both. The conclusion that 'a person is not necessarily responsible for someone else's needing to be saved; but he is responsible for anyone he kills' (ibid.) is thus false, morally irrelevant, or ambiguous, depending on whether 'responsibility' refers to causal or moral responsibility throughout, or whether Trammel means 'moral responsibility' in one place and 'causal responsibility' in the other. See also Bruce Russell: 'On the Relative Strictness of Negative and Positive Duties', in Steinbock (ed.): *Killing and Letting Die*, 222-4.

[92] See also Russell: 'On the Relative Strictness', 223.

*Y* subsequently to die of the disease, I would be 'more morally responsible' for *Y*'s death than the doctor who refrained from preventing *Y*'s death. The converse is the case.

I take it, then, that neither Green nor Trammel has shown that an agent who initiates a course of events that will lead to death is morally more responsible for the resultant death than an agent who refrains from intervening in a causal process not of her making, foreseeing that her non-intervention will result in a preventable death.

### 2.72   *The Presumption of Knowing What is Best and Optionality*

Are there any other reasons for thinking that the distinction between killing and letting die, or between positive and negative euthanasia, has intrinsic moral significance? Trammel advances another argument designed to show that positive and negative euthanasia differ in the likelihood of certain serious errors, and with regard to the presumption that we know what is best for a patient:

> ... there are morally relevant differences between positive and negative ... euthanasia ... negative euthanasia is more easily justified than positive euthanasia. Positive euthanasia, by its external inducement to death, involves the risk of certain types of serious error which negative euthanasia does not involve. Positive euthanasia drastically cuts off options to help the person in unanticipated ways which negative euthanasia leaves open. An active attempt to kill a person for that person's sake involves the presumption that we know what is best for that person, whereas not administering certain treatment does not necessarily involve such a presumption.[93]

It is obvious, though, that negative euthanasia cannot be distinguished from positive euthanasia on the grounds that the latter does, but the former does not, involve the presumption that the agent knows what is best for a patient. Whilst it is generally true that a doctor does not give a lethal injection unless she believes that it is in the patient's best interest not to survive, it is also true that a doctor does not generally refrain from preventing death unless she believes that it is in the patient's best interest not to have her life prolonged. We can kill or let die for any number of reasons, one of which is the presumption that we know what is best for a person. The *method*, killing or letting die, is irrelevant as far as that issue is concerned.

It is, of course, true that a doctor can sometimes, as Trammel says, 'not administer certain treatment' without thereby refraining from

[93] Richard R. Trammel: 'The Presumption against Taking Life', *The Journal of Medicine and Philosophy* 3 (1978), 63.

preventing death when, for example, she does not know what kind of treatment might, under the circumstances, be effective; when certain kinds of treatment are simply not available, or when the patient refuses further medical intervention. In all these cases, a doctor is, however, not *refraining* from preventing a patient's death; and we cannot use these instances to distinguish killing from letting die, or positive from negative euthanasia.

Similarly Trammel's second point. The difference between positive and negative euthanasia does not lie in the fact that positive euthanasia cuts off options that negative euthanasia leaves open.

From the *result* perspective, killing and letting die are the same. In both cases, death is a necessary condition for a killing or a letting die to have taken place. And from the *decision* perspective, death is not a necessary condition for either an attempted killing or an attempted letting die.[94] It is a matter of probabilities. And, as far as probabilities are concerned, it may even be the case that the probability of death is greater when an agent decides to refrain from saving than when she decides to kill. (Compare my attempting to kill you by shooting over a distance of three hundred metres and your refraining from pulling me back into the boat after I have fallen into piranha-infested waters three hundred metres from shore.) If, as we have seen in Section 2.2, all untreated spina bifida infants in one non-treatment regime die within the first four weeks of life, no options are left open. This means that if the aim were to leave options open, then not only positive but also negative euthanasia would have to be prohibited.

## 2.73  Dischargeability of Duties

Trammel points out correctly that given the world as it is, it is impossible for one person 'to aid everyone who needs help'. Yet it is possible to refrain from killing and harming people. This is so because 'refraining from the action of killing is a kind of "inaction" ... Saving is a kind of "action" ...' Since positive actions usually require effort whereas refrainings do not, denial of a morally relevant distinction between the two 'leads straight to an ethic so strenuous that it might give pause even to a philosophical John the Baptist'.[95] The point underlying Trammel's analysis, which he explores in terms

---

[94] Morillo: 'Doing, Refraining', 36.
[95] Trammel: 'Saving Life and Taking Life', 131–3.

of 'negative' versus 'positive duties' (or the duty to refrain from killing versus the duty to positively save a person), appears to be this:

Inaction involves allowing the flow of events to move in the direction it is moving, without our intervention. Thus inaction is essentially related to lack of effort. Action involves changing the flow of events from the direction in which it would flow without our intervention. This is another reason the distinction between action and inaction has intrinsic moral relevance.[96]

However, as I have argued throughout this chapter, killing and letting die cannot be distinguished in terms of action or inaction. Nor can they be distinguished in terms of effort required to change the flow of events from the direction in which it would move without our intervention. The latter point is illustrated by the following example:

One person spends an hour putting up a bird house which helps to bring about the successful nesting of bluebirds (who are not doing so well these days). Another discovers bluebirds nesting at the hinge of his closed garage door. Rather than disturb the birds, he leaves his car in the garage for the duration of the nesting period, at considerable personal inconvenience.[97]

There is no general rule that 'making happen' requires more effort than 'letting happen'. It is true that refraining from killing generally requires less effort than saving someone's life. But even if this is true, it does, of course, not show that killing is worse than letting die.

This can be seen most clearly when we consider the following point. Trammel holds that 'euthanasia must be for the sake of the person who dies';[98] but if this is the case, then the notions of harming and benefiting interwoven with Trammel's distinction between positive and negative duties are reversed in cases of euthanasia, and applied differently from the way in which they are normally applied to what we do to our fellow human beings. While death is normally an evil, and to kill a person is harming her, this is not the case in euthanasia as understood by Trammel. In all these cases where euthanasia is justified, death is positively valued end from the patient's point of view; to kill or let die is thus not harming the patient, but benefiting her. But if death is a benefit to the patient, and by implication continued life a harm, then—surely—to kill a patient (and to positively benefit her) is not worse (and may be better) than merely

---

[96] Trammel: 'The Presumption against Taking Life', 65.
[97] Morillo: 'Doing, Refraining', 36.
[98] See Trammel: 'The Presumption against Taking Life', 56.

allowing benefit to befall her. Thus even if there were an asymmetry between positive and negative duties, it does not follow that killing is intrinsically worse than letting die.[99]

## 2.74   The Residual Difference: 'Making Happen' and 'Letting Happen'

Ultimately, analyses like those of Trammel, Green, and many others seem to hinge on the residual difference between killing and letting die previously identified: killing and letting die can be distinguished in so far as they involve the agent at different stages of a causal chain—and in the medical setting, generally in different causal chains. The patient's death will either be a consequence of a disease, or a consequence of a lethal agent administered by the doctor.

In the previously cited quote, Mill points out that 'many causes may produce death'.[100] And, building on Mill, Mackie draws our attention to the fact that there are many minimally sufficient conditions for a consequence such as death. The act of killing a patient by a lethal injection is an *inus* condition in one minimally sufficient condition for death, and hence a cause of death; refraining from administering a life-saving course of antibiotics to a patient who is suffering from, say, pneumonia, is an *inus* condition in another minimally sufficient condition for death, and hence another cause. Whilst these two modes of causing death cannot be distinguished in terms of causal efficacy or in terms of causal agency, they can be distinguished in so far as in the first case the physician *initiates* a course of events that will lead to death, whereas in the second case the doctor *refrains from intervening* in a course of events not initiated by her that will, coupled with her refraining, also lead to the patient's death.

However, why should the mere distinction between 'making happen' and 'letting happen' make a difference if all other morally relevant factors are the same? To show why people might hold this view, let me once again quote Vincent J. Collins, a doctor, this time at some greater length:

A physician's approach to the inevitable ending of life may be either passive

---

[99] See also Holly Goldman: 'Killing, Letting Die and Euthanasia', *Analysis* 40 (1980) 224; Natalie Abrams: 'Active and Passive Euthanasia', *Philosophy* 53 (1978), 257–63. For two arguments that our positive duty to save is no less stringent than our negative duty not to kill, see James Rachels: 'Killing and Starving to Death', *Philosophy* 54 (1979), 159–71; and Russell: 'On the Relative Strictness', 215–31.

[100] See n. 54.

or active. Death could occur by actively interceding or by passively discontinuing therapy. In the first instance, one directly causes life to end by an overt act, whereas by discontinuing therapy, one permits death to occur by omitting to act and permitting nature to take its course.

When one actively intercedes, one is, in fact, causing harm to the individual, even though this harm may apparently have a good intent; here man is acting . . . Shall we perform a deliberate act to positively end life? From the legal standpoint, from the moral codes, and from the guidelines of medical practice we find applied the general law that one is not permitted to actively kill . . . regardless of intent . . . But we must distinguish clearly between letting a patient die and euthanasia . . . When one permits death by not continuing therapy, the harm that is done is done by nature acting. This is passive management based on reason and judgment—and shortening the act of dying. It is rational.[101]

Whilst I do not want to impute the views advanced by Collins to either Green or Trammel, both seem to agree with Collins on one point: we are fully responsible for what we 'make happen' and somewhat less responsible for what we 'let happen'. But why, one might ask, should anyone regard the distinction between 'making happen' and 'letting happen' as morally relevant in itself?

It may be that the view that we are 'more responsible' for the consequences of a causal process initiated by us than we are for the consequences of a causal process not of our making rests ultimately on nothing more substantial that the doubtful metaphysical assumption (almost explicit in Collins) that Nature (or God?) is the dominant agent, and that in refraining from preventing death an agent merely lets happen what Nature brings about.[102] In letting die, an agent does thus not 'make it happen' that death occurs, she merely refrains from preventing its occurrence; and in merely 'letting happen', she does not positively shape the course of events—she does not 'play God', but rather leaves it up to God, or Nature, whether, and if so when, a consequence such as death will occur.

To subscribe to such a view of agency is, however, an abdication of moral responsibility and a stance that leads, as we shall see, to decision-making being based on morally irrelevant grounds. Moreover, it is conceptually flawed: we are just as responsible, both causally and morally, for what we let happen as we are for what we make happen, all else being equal.

[101] Collins: 'Limits of Medical Responsibility', 390.
[102] See also D. N. Walton: *On Defining Depth* (Montreal: McGill–Queen's University Press, 1979). 118–20.

Does this mean, then, that the qualified Sanctity-of-Life Principle is untenable and ought to be rejected? Before we can answer that question, we need to examine the other two major distinctions adduced to support the qualified SLP: the distinction between what an agent intends and what she foresees, and the distinction between ordinary and extraordinary means of treatment. I shall examine these in Chapters 3 and 4, respectively.

# 3

# The Intentional Termination of Life and the Principle of Double Effect

There is a further clear distinction between using means for the relief of suffering which may, as a secondary result, shorten life, and actively ending life. Here the guide is the principle known as the principle of double effect. It is as a principle commonly misunderstood, but one which in fact guides doctors whenever the problem of undesirable side-effects arises with any treatment. . . . The use of medicaments with the intention of relieving pain is good, and if by repeated pain relief the patient's resistance is lowered and he dies earlier than he would otherwise have done, this is a side-effect which may well be acceptable. . . . On the other hand, to give an overdose *with the intention that the patient should never wake up* is morally wrong. It is killing.

> Jonathan Gould *et al.*: *Your Death Warrant? The Implications of Euthanasia*

It is altogether too artificial to say that a doctor who gives an overdose of a narcotic having in the forefront of his mind the aim of ending the patient's existence is guilty of sin, while a doctor who gives the same overdose in the same circumstances in order to relieve pain is not guilty of sin, provided he keeps his mind off the consequence which his professional training teaches him is inevitable, namely, the death of his patient. . . . If The Doctrine of Double Effect means that the necessity of making a choice of values can be avoided merely by keeping your mind off one of the consequences, it can only encourage a hypocritical attitude towards moral problems.

> Glanville Williams: *The Sanctity of Life and the Criminal Law*

## 3.1 INTRODUCTION: ABSOLUTISM AND THE PRINCIPLE OF DOUBLE EFFECT

As we saw in Chapter 2, when a doctor refrains from preventing a patient's death, her refraining is a cause of that patient's death; moreover, I argued, the doctor is not only causally but also prima facie morally responsible for the patient's death—just as responsible as she would have been had she administered a lethal injection. If the Sanctity-of-Life Principle were thus to prohibit a doctor from ever voluntarily and deliberately causing death, then not only killing but also allowing to die would be completely ruled out, and consistency would demand that every life that can be prolonged would have to be prolonged by all available means. And yet, doctors do not prolong the lives of all patients. We have, for example, already seen that it is common medical practice to let some seriously handicapped infants die. In this and subsequent chapters, we shall also encounter examples of deliberate lettings die in other areas of medicine.

Are doctors, then, in deliberately allowing some of their patients to die, infringing the sanctity-of-life doctrine? Not necessarily so. There may be another way of making the qualified SLP consistent—namely, by showing that a distinction can be drawn, in terms of the agent's intention between permissible and impermissible instances of causing a patient's death.

What is clear, then, is this: to be consistent, the qSLP must regard some instances of an agent voluntarily causing death as not being instances of the *intentional* causation of death. For if an agent could be said intentionally to bring about all the foreseen consequences of her deliberate and voluntary actions or omissions, then the qSLP would be glaringly inconsistent: on this broad conception of the intentional, the qSLP would both prohibit and permit the intentional causation of death.

The qualified SLP thus rests on there being a coherent, narrower conception of the intentional. This, supporters of the SLP say, is found in the distinction between those consequences which an agent desires, aims at, or wants, and those which she merely foresees but does not desire or want. In other words, a distinction is drawn between the 'directly intended' and the 'merely foreseen' consequences of an agent's action or omission.

This distinction between 'directly intended' and 'merely foreseen' consequences of an action or omission is thus of great importance to supporters of the sanctity-of-life view. It would counter the devastating charge of formal inconsistency, and would also avoid the counterintuitive implication that a doctor must always sustain a patient's life by all available means.

Many of the actual rulings made by supporters of the SLP are based on such a narrow conception of the intentional. The Vatican's

*Declaration on Euthanasia*, for example, allows not only that a doctor may sometimes withhold or withdraw life-sustaining treatment, but also that she may administer a potentially lethal dose of narcotics in order to alleviate the patient's pain, even if it is foreseen that her doing so will bring about the patient's death. In this case, the *Declaration* says, 'death is in no way intended or sought, even if the risk of it is reasonably taken'.[1] To perform intentionally a good or morally indifferent action (for example, relieve pain) that is believed to also bring about death, or to refrain from employing life-prolonging treatment so as not to prolong the patient's suffering is, on this view, not the intentional termination of life, and hence permissible.

The distinction between intended results and foreseen but non-intended further consequences is formalized in the Principle of Double Effect (hereafter 'PDE'), to be discussed in detail in Section 3.2. The PDE figures prominently in many non-consequentialist ethics, but is of special importance for absolutist moral schemes which hold that certain kinds of action are not only intrinsically but *absolutely* wrong, whatever the consequences of not performing the prohibited action. The PDE has thus long been an important element of Catholic moral thinking.[2] In recent years, however, the application of this principle has not been limited to either Catholics or theologians, and the PDE, or propositions having close affinities with it, have aroused considerable philosophical interest.[3] This interest has primarily focused on the distinction drawn by the PDE between intended and merely foreseen consequences of an agent's deliberate action or omission. That these distinctions have often focused on the morality of killing is not surprising. It is not only that the intentional termination of innocent human lives is perhaps the most widely accepted moral prohibition; it is also that in two different areas—war and the practice of medicine—it has become increasingly difficult to maintain that some accepted practices do not constitute the intentional termination of innocent human lives. Modern science and

---

[1] Sacred Congregation: *Declaration on Euthanasia*, 8–9.

[2] See Joseph Mangan: 'An Historical Analysis of the Principle of Double Effect', *Theological Studies* 10 (1949), 41–61.

[3] See, for example, Bennett: 'Whatever the Consequences', 211–36; Foot: 'Abortion and Double Effect', 156–65; L. W. Sumner: *Abortion and Moral Theory* (Princeton: Princeton University Press, 1981), 115–23; Glover: *Causing Death and Saving Lives*, 86–91; Charles Fried: *Right and Wrong* (Cambridge, Mass.: Harvard University Press, 1978), 20–8.

technology have sharpened the focus, not by creating problems that are entirely new but by portraying old practical and philosophical problems with greater clarity and urgency. In war, powerful new weapons do not selectively kill combatants, leaving the 'innocent' unharmed; rather, they kill combatants and non-combatants alike. This means that those who want to uphold the absolute prohibition against the intentional killing of the innocent must either abandon modern modes of waging war (and of thus defending certain values) or if they don't, they must find means of distinguishing—in terms of the agent's intention, rather than in terms of foreseen consequences— between prohibited and permissible instances of an agent voluntarily and deliberately taking innocent human lives.[4]

In the practice of medicine, we have analogous developments. Powerful narcotics, not generally available until the end of the nineteenth century and not well understood in their efficacy until the present one, can alleviate pain that could formerly not be alleviated. They kill not only the pain, but—if given in increasingly large doses— also the patient. If a doctor thus administers what she believes to be a lethal dose of a pain-killing drug, she has initiated a causal process that is, under the circumstances, sufficient to cause the patient's death. If the patient dies, then her death is the result of a killing. Again, those who want to uphold the absolute prohibition against intentionally killing the innocent, whilst also wanting to allow the alleviation of pain with sufficiently large doses of drugs, must attempt to distinguish in terms of the agent's intention, rather than in terms of foreseen consequences, between permissible and prohibited instances of an agent doing something that she believes will inevitably or very likely result in the death of an innocent human being.

Similarly in the case of a doctor refraining from prolonging life. Modern medical science and technology have made it possible to prolong the lives of many patients, even in situations where the prolongation of such lives would also constitute the prolongation of great suffering. In Chapter 2, we briefly looked at the selective non-treatment of infants afflicted with severe forms of spina bifida. Most of these infants would have died in earlier times when modern medical technology was not available to keep them alive. Today this technology is available. If a doctor refrains from using it—that is, if

---

[4] See, for example, G. E. M. Anscombe: 'War and Murder', in R. Wasserstrom (ed.): *War and Morality* (Belmont: Wadsworth, 1970), 42–53; Thomas Nagel: 'War and Massacre', *Philosophy and Public Affairs* (1972), 123–44.

she does not operate, use antibiotics, and so on, and believes that death will occur as a consequence of her omission—she lets the patient die. Is this an instance of the intentional termination of life, or a permissible instance of allowing death to occur?

According to most defenders of the SLP, neither 'pyramid' pain-killing (i.e. the administration of increasing and finally lethal doses of pain-killing drugs), nor the withholding or withdrawing of life-prolonging treatment is under certain conditions (to be discussed in subsequent sections of this chapter) the intentional termination of life. If, under those circumstances, a doctor merely foresees that death will occur as a consequence of what she intentionally does without also aiming at, or intending, the patient's death, then (so the argument goes) she does not infringe the absolute prohibition against the intentional termination of life.

This is so, a defender of absolute prohibitions, such as Charles Fried, will argue, because the intrinsic wrongness of killing lies in 'what it is wrong to do', where the principles' absolute force 'attaches only to what we intend, and not to the whole range of things which come about as a result of what we do intentionally'. As long as the bad effect, death, is neither aimed at as an end, nor chosen as a means to an end, but is merely permitted to come about, an agent has not done what it is absolutely wrong to do.[5]

The absolutist SLP thus prohibits not killing and letting die *as such*: rather, it prohibits the intentional termination of innocent human lives, either positively or negatively. As R. A. Duff puts it:

The absolutist . . . is primarily concerned with the intentional actions of human agents, rather than their consequences. What matters is not simply that an event occurs which I did, or could, foresee and control, but the way in which I am related, as an agent, to that event: what matters is what I *do*; and 'what I do' is determined not just by what happens, but by the intention revealed in my action . . . His absolute prohibition is against the intentional action of killing, not against the occurrence of the foreseen and avoidable causation of death: it would indeed be absurd to prohibit *that* absolutely, since for any prohibited outcome we could imagine a case in which the outcome of any alternative is even worse.[6]

What is important for the absolutist, Duff continues, is to give a clear account of the notion of agency: 'to show the sense that it has, in

[5] Fried: *Right and Wrong*, 20–1.
[6] R. A. Duff: 'Absolute Principles and Double Effect', *Analysis* 36, (1976), 74.

particular contexts, and to show how it is part of an intelligible moral perspective of human life'.

This task, Duff holds, is facilitated by the fact that also 'we', who are not all absolutists, attribute a similar significance to human agency:

We draw moral distinctions between what we intentionally do and what our actions foreseeably cause or what we fail to prevent; between the harm we intentionally cause and that which we fail to avert or which occurs as a by-product of some other intentional action; between trying to harm someone and recognizing that he will or may be injured by what we do: and we may sometimes allow the one while condemning the other.[7]

In so far as Duff is concerned with the explication of the PDE and the intention/foresight distinction, the crucial difference between the intentional and the non-intentional termination of life lies thus not in the end-result—the occurrence of a foreseen and preventable death— but in the agent's intention in relation to the death; death must not be the direct object of the agent's will.[8]

The claim that a clear conceptual and moral distinction exists between what we intentionally bring about and what we merely allow to happen has, in many cases, an initial intuitive plausibility. Philippa Foot tries to illustrate this intuitive distinction in the following way. She says,

Most of us allow people to die of starvation in India and Africa, and there is surely something wrong with us that we do; it would be nonsense, however, to pretend that it is only in law that we make a distinction between allowing people in the underdeveloped countries to die of starvation and sending them poisoned food.[9]

The initial plausibility of examples such as these rests, however, on an inappropriate characterization of the intention/foresight distinction. As the example stands, poisoning and allowing to die are not instances of an agent deliberately bringing about both a good and a bad effect. This means that the Principle of Double Effect can not even begin to be applied. In addition to that, we would expect that differences in certainty of outcome, motivation, and so on, would account for the intuitive plausibility of the claim that poisoning is, in

---

[7] Ibid.

[8] In the above quotation, Duff is, in fact, appealing to a number of different distinctions (e.g. acts and omissions, trying to harm and allowing harm to occur), which are not identical with the intention/foresight distinction. See also Sect. 3.6.

[9] Foot: 'Abortion and Double Effect', 161–2.

this case, worse than letting die. What is at issue, though, is not the killing/letting die distinction as such, nor the question whether killing is often worse than letting die; rather, what is at issue is whether a morally relevant distinction can be drawn between what an agent intends and what she foresees—that is, between what are regarded as clear examples of intentional and non-intentional killings on the one hand, and intentional and non-intentional lettings die on the other—when all other things are equal.

Here it is important to note three distinctions—already recognized by Jeremy Bentham—between those consequences that

1. we intend as our ends (or for their own sake);
2. those that we intend as means to our further ends; and
3. consequences that occur as side-effects or further consequences of what we do intentionally.[10]

Bentham is in agreement with supporters of the SLP when he suggests that an agent 'directly' intends not only her actual end, but also whatever she chooses as a means to that end, although she only 'obliquely intends' (a supporter of the SLP would want to say 'foresees', 'allows', or 'permits') a certain secondary effect. This tripartite distinction, to which I shall return in more detail below, raises not one question, but two:

1. Can a coherent and morally relevant distinction be drawn between those consequences that are 'intended as means' and those consequences that are 'obliquely intended'?
2. Can a coherent and morally relevant distinction be drawn between what an agent intends as her end and what she either intends as a means or brings about as a side-effect or further consequence of what she does?

I shall argue, in Sections 3.2–3.6, that actual rulings made by supporters of the SLP on the basis of the PDE, or of propositions having close affinities with it, do not allow us to distinguish—in terms of the agent's intention—between permissible and impermissible instances of bringing about a death, or of allowing a death to occur. Moreover, I shall argue, particularly in Sections 3.3 and 3.6, that theories espoused by supporters of the SLP make the distinction between 'means' and 'side-effects' as per (1) above highly problematic. I shall argue further that the distinction as per (2) between 'ends',

[10] Bentham: *Principles of Morals and Legislation*, Chs. 8, 9, 82–96.

and 'means' or 'side-effects'—to the extent that it can be drawn—involves a confusion between the nature of *actions* and the goodness or badness of *agents* (Section 3.6).

As a corollary of the above, the narrow conception of the intentional becomes untenable. This leaves us, in the absence of a plausible 'intermediary' theory, with the broad conception of the intentional according to which an agent intends all the foreseen consequences of her actions or omissions. But, as we have already seen in Section 1.6, this broad conception of the intentional is incompatible with absolute moral rules, and would make the unqualified or 'pure' SLP unintelligible. The SLP would be unintelligible because it would, in conflict situations, require incompatible actions: for example, it might require us to save the lives of five by killing one, whilst also requiring us to let five die by refraining from killing one.

## 3.2    THE PRINCIPLE OF DOUBLE EFFECT, ABORTION, AND THE PROBLEM OF INTENTION

### *3.21    The Principle of Double Effect: Introduction*

Supporters of the Sanctity-of-Life Principle have traditionally appealed to the Principle of Double Effect (PDE), so as to maintain the absolute prohibition against the intentional termination of innocent human life in the face of situations which seem to reduce the SLP to absurdity because so obviously contrary to other values, including the value of human life. The PDE defines those conditions under which agents may *bring about* death, or *allow* death to occur, as a secondary effect of some morally good (or at least morally indifferent) action or omission.

Whilst the PDE has thus long been a mainstem of Thomistic moral theology, philosophical interest in it has undoubtedly been motivated by two quite different factors. Those with leanings towards a deontological view of morality have argued that the doctrine's central distinction between what a person foresees and what, in the narrow sense, she intends is essential to any satisfactory discussion of agency and its implications for the general issue of killing and of its particular aspects, such as abortion, infanticide, euthanasia, and so on.[11] And

---

[11] See, e.g., Foot: 'Abortion and Double Effect', 156–65. Philip E. Devine: *The Ethics of Homicide* (Ithaca: Cornell University Press, 1978), 106–26; Fried: *Right and Wrong*, 20–8; Thomas Nagel: 'The Limits of Objectivity', in McMurrin (ed.): *The Tanner Lectures*, vol. i, 76–139.

on the other hand, those tending towards a more consequentialist view of morality have argued that the SLP, coupled with the PDE, has unacceptable moral consequences: it allows doctors to bring about the death of their patients by either pyramid pain-killing or the slow process of withholding life-sustaining treatment, whilst never permitting that a doctor directly terminate a patient's life—thus condoning more rather than less suffering, on the basis of a distinction that is, in itself, morally irrelevant.[12]

What, then, are the conditions under which an agent may bring about a bad effect, or allow a bad effect to occur? The PDE outlines four conditions, and the *New Catholic Encyclopaedia* lists these as follows:

1. The act itself must be morally good, or at least indifferent.
2. The agent may not positively will the bad effect but may permit it. If he could attain the good effect without the bad effect he should do so. The bad effect is sometimes said to be indirectly voluntary.
3. The good effect must flow from the action at least as immediately (in order of causality, though not necessarily in the order of time) as the bad effect. In other words, the good effect must be produced directly by the action, not by the bad effect. Otherwise the agent would be using a bad means to a good end, which is never allowed.
4. The good effect must be sufficiently desirable to compensate for the allowing of the bad effect. In forming this decision many factors must be weighed and compared, with care and prudence proportionate to the importance of the case . . .[13]

The PDE thus stipulates that a bad effect, such as the death of an innocent human being, is sometimes 'allowed' or 'permitted' to occur, although it must not be intended by the agent. Here it should be emphasized that the distinction drawn by the PDE between the intentional and the non-intentional termination of life is not the distinction between killing and letting die. According to Thomistic moral theology, in which the PDE is said to have had its origin,[14] a person can kill another without intending her death; and, on the other

[12] See, e.g., James Rachels: 'Active and Passive Euthanasia', in Steinbock (ed.): *Killing and Letting Die*, 63–8; Michael Tooley: 'An Irrelevant Consideration: Killing versus Letting Die', ibid., 56–62; Harris: *Violence and Responsibility*, 48–65.

[13] Catholic University of America, *New Catholic Encyclopaedia*, vol. 4 (New York: McGraw Hill, 1976), 1020–22.

[14] See, e.g., Germain Grisez: 'Toward a Consistent Natural Law Ethics of Killing', *American Journal of Jurisprudence* 15 (1970), 64–96. Grisez suggests that the PDE has its origin in Thomas Aquinas's justification of killing in self-defence. (See Sect. 3.3 for a discussion of self-defence in the context of abortion.)

hand, intend the death of someone whom she lets die. What Thomism—and the SLP— thus prohibit is the intentional termination of life, be this an instance of killing or of letting die.

In this connection, we should note a further point: whilst the PDE is made necessary by particular moral systems based on exceptionless moral rules, which create the need for guidance in conflict situations, it is not identical with absolutism.[15] Contrary to some interpretations, the PDE does not stipulate that it is, for example, always absolutely prohibited intentionally to terminate innocent human life, nor does the PDE explain how one is to arrive at the normative judgements presupposed by the first three conditions, which characterize an act as morally good. Similarly the bad effect: the PDE does not explain which effects are bad and why. This means that any moral theory which holds that some acts are intrinsically good or bad, simply in virtue of the kinds of act they are, would be consistent with the PDE and could employ it in conflict situations.

But if the PDE is not identical with absolutism, this means that some of the criticisms levelled against the principle are misdirected. H. L. A. Hart, for example, discusses the following case:

A man was trapped in the cabin of a blazing lorry, with no hope of being freed. He asked a bystander to shoot him in order to save him from further agony. The bystander did so. Hart thinks the PDE 'would forbid what was done in this case',[16] and he urges that the principle be rejected because it leads to morally unacceptable conclusions.

The point, however, is that the intentional killing of the trapped man is condemned not by the PDE but by those moralities which regard the intentional termination of innocent human life as absolutely wrong—for example, Catholic moral theology, or the sanctity-of-life doctrine. If the PDE is applied in the context of an absolutist morality that prohibits the intentional termination of life, then it may well rule as Hart thinks it would. But if it does, then the *source* of that counter-intuitive ruling lies not in the PDE but in exceptionless moral prohibitions.

---

[15] See, e.g., Sumner: *Abortion and Moral Theory*, 115–16. Sumner assumes that the PDE is firmly linked to absolutism: 'The intrinsic quality-condition presupposes that certain acts are absolutely impermissible simply in virtue of the kinds of acts they are.' However, what the PDE presupposes is not the absolute impermissibility of performing certain acts, but rather that there are some acts which are intrinsically wrong.

[16] Hart: 'Intention and Punishment', in Hart: *Punishment and Responsibility*, 123.

## 3.22   When is Death Intended?

For the purposes of this book, I shall primarily be concerned with the application of the PDE within the absolutist perspective of the sanctity-of-life doctrine. Application of the PDE presupposes that the principle is intelligible, and that its central distinction—that between intention and foresight—can satisfactorily be drawn. But, as we shall see, this distinction is problematic.

There are serious philosophical problems in any systematic application of the concept of intention, and the literature is replete with criticisms and refutations. The notion underlying the PDE is stated in conditions 2 and 3. However, in the absence of a fuller account of the concept of intention, its characterization as that which an agent 'positively wills', either as her chosen end or as a means to her end, is not very helpful in many difficult cases. Whilst it is, in many cases, intuitively obvious when an agent can be said to have intended a bad effect, there are other cases where it is not. Cases such as the following have been adduced to point out this difficulty:

A party of explorers is trapped in a cave, in whose narrow opening a rather fat member of the party is lodged, and the waters are rising. If a member of the party explodes a charge next to the fat man, should we say that he intended the fat man's death as a means or that it is a mere side effect of (*a*) freeing the party, (*b*) removing the fat man's body from the opening, or most implausibly, (*c*) blowing him to atoms?[17]

In cases such as these, it might be thought that the official rulings of the PDE might throw some light on what conditions must be fulfilled for an agent to have positively willed a bad effect either as her end or as a means to it. As we shall see, though, the most plausible interpretations of the second and third conditions of the PDE appear not to support the actual judgements purportedly made on the basis of them.

### 3.23   The Problem with Abortion

Since the PDE has received its most thorough discussion in connection with the problem of abortion, I shall initially focus on abortion as an example of the application of this principle to the distinction between intentional and non-intentional killings.

Within the sanctity-of-life doctrine, the prohibition of abortion follows from the acceptance of the prohibition against the intentional

[17] Fried: *Right and Wrong*, 23.

taking of innocent human life and from the premiss that an innocent human being exists from the moment of conception. I will analyse two frequently discussed cases involving the death of a foetus, where the PDE is said to permit bringing about the foetus's death in the first case but not in the second case. As we shall see, though, the problem of intention remains unresolved.

> *Case A*: A pregnant woman has a cancerous uterus. If the cancer is not removed, both the woman and the foetus will die. If the cancer is removed, the woman will be saved. The only way to completely remove the cancer is to perform a hysterectomy—resulting in the foetus's certain death.
>
> *Case B*: A woman suffering from a serious heart condition becomes pregnant. Both the woman and the foetus will die unless the foetus is removed at an early stage of pregnancy. An early abortion will save the mother's life, but will result in the foetus's certain death.[18]

Both the hysterectomy in Case *A* and the abortion in Case *B* are actions of double effect: both have the good effect of saving the woman's life and the bad effect of also bringing about the death of the foetus. However, whilst it is traditionally assumed that the PDE will permit bringing about the death of the foetus in Case *A*, the same tradition holds that it will not permit the abortion in Case *B*. Since the two cases are parallel as far as the good effect (saving the woman's life) and the bad effect (death of the foetus) are concerned, they cannot be distinguished by way of the PDE's proportionality criterion (condition 4). It would therefore appear that what distinguishes these two cases must be the agent's intention revealed by her action. To remove the foetus in Case *B* is regarded as an instance of the intentional termination of life; to remove the cancerous womb and the foetus in Case *A* is not.[19]

Let us see whether the claim can be supported that the agent in Case *B* does, and the agent in Case *A* does not, intend to produce the foetus's death.

The notion of what either agent can be said to intend must have a weaker sense than that given by 'pursue as an end'—that is, as

[18] See Sumner: *Abortion and Moral Theory*, 115–23, for a discussion of a similar set of examples; also S. M. Uniacke: 'The Doctrine of Double Effect', *The Thomist* 48: 2 (April 1984), 188–218.

[19] See Pius XII, Address to the Catholic Society of Midwives, 29 October 1951, *Acta Apostolicae Sedis* 43, (1951), 838 ff; see also Kelly: *Medico-moral Problems*, 62–9.

something pursued or sought for its own sake; for neither agent need regard the foetus's death as intrinsically desirable. On the other hand, it must be a stronger sense than 'foreseen as an inevitable or highly likely consequence of one's conduct', for both agents foresee the death of the foetus.

The standard account is that the two cases are distinguishable on the grounds that the death of the foetus in Case *B* is a *means* to saving the woman's life (see clause 3 of the PDE), whereas it is merely a foreseen secondary effect of what the agent does in the Case of *A*. Chosen means, it is held, are as much intended as one's chosen objectives. Since the death of the foetus in Case *B* is a means to saving the woman's life, its death must be intended: it is an instance of intentional killing. As Elizabeth Anscome puts it in a related context: 'It is nonsense to pretend that you do not intend to do what is the means you take to your chosen end.'[20]

This needs explication and explanation. Here I shall briefly state the issues, which will occupy us for much of this chapter.

The distinction between means and ends, and the claim that we must intend to do what are the means to our chosen ends, derives its intuitive plausibility from the distinction between what, for example, Jeremy Bentham calls 'ultimately' and 'mediately' intentional incidents in one chain of motives. Bentham illustrates this distinction by two possible interpretations of Sir Walter Tyrrell's lethally wounding William II whilst on a stag hunt:

1. He [Tyrrell] killed the king on account of the hatred he bore him, and for no other reason than the pleasure of destroying him. In this case the king's death was not only directly but also ultimately intentional.
2. He [Tyrrell] killed the king intending fully so to do; not for any hatred he bore him but for the sake of plundering him when dead. In this case the incident of the king's death was directly intentional, but not ultimately: it was mediately intentional.[21]

In Case 2 we can apparently clearly distinguish between means and ends, and there seems to be little doubt that Tyrrell intended to do what was the means (killing the king) to his chosen end (plundering the king). But this simplicity is deceptive and two questions are raised immediately. Firstly, did Tyrrell intend to *kill* the king (or only render him inoperative so that he could plunder him) and, secondly, whether

---

[20] Anscombe: 'War and Murder', 51.
[21] Bentham: *Principles of Morals and Legislation*, 84–6; see also n. 10.

the distinction between means and ends—here drawn between *two* distinct actions (killing and plundering)—can also be drawn within a *single* human action whose nature is said to be determined by what the agent intends. The first question will be discussed in the present section, the second in Section 3.3.

In Case *B*, we have a single action that has both a good and a bad effect, and we might begin by asking in what sense the *death* of the foetus can be regarded as a necessary means to saving the mother's life. Surely, as in Case *A*, it is not the foetus's death that is necessary for saving the mother—only its *removal* from her body is. Why, then, we might ask, is it held that the agent in Case *A* does not, but the agent in Case *B* does, intend the foetus's death? After all, the foetus is *removed* from the woman's body in either case—the only difference being that in one case the foetus is removed together with the womb, whereas in the other it is removed without the womb.

In this connection, also condition 2 of the PDE is of importance. Condition 2 requires that the agent bring about the good effect without the bad where this is possible. This stipulation would initially appear to be of great importance for the determination of intention, and it has given rise to a traditional criterion, the counter-factual test: if the bad effect could somehow be prevented, and if events thereafter were allowed to take their 'natural' course, would the agent still have chosen to act the way she did? For example, if an abortion could be performed in such a way that it did not entail the death of the foetus, and if the foetus could then be kept alive outside the womb, would the agent choose the non-lethal mode of procuring the abortion? If such available options were not chosen, then it would be difficult to argue that the death of the foetus was not intended.

Philippa Foot, in her discussion of the PDE, makes a similar point. She cites the previously encountered example of a runaway tram which the driver can only steer from one narrow tunnelled track to another. If the driver stays on the same track, five men will be killed. If he changes to the other track, one man will be killed. Does the driver when changing tracks intend the one man's death? No, says Foot. For if the man were miraculously to survive by, say, clinging on to the side of the tunnel, 'the driver of the tram does not then leap off and brain him with a crowbar'. This shows, Foot says, that the driver does not intend the man's death; he merely allows it to occur.[22]

Whilst this test for establishing an agent's intention may be helpful

[22] Foot: 'Abortion and Double Effect', 159.

in some cases, it seems to allow far more than its proponents are willing to grant. Take another of Foot's examples—the judicial execution of one innocent man to save five others, which she contrasts with that of the runaway tram. She suggests that we would be appalled at the framing of the innocent man, for in this case the judge 'aims' at the innocent man's death as 'part of his plan'.[23] But even here, the distinction Foot wants to draw between an agent aiming/not aiming at another person's death is not clear. If we understand an execution as *logically* entailing the death of an innocent man, then we might say that his death must be intended. But we need not understand the framing of the innocent man in this way: if the judge could somehow create the appearance of the man's death without actually having him killed, then he would, we assume, not ensure that the man dies some other way.

Similarly the example of the fat man stuck in the cave. If, by some remote chance, the fat man survived being dynamited out of the hole, his friends—just like the driver of the runaway tram—would not then brain him with a crowbar. The same considerations hold in the case of Abortion *B*. Whilst this abortion would initially seem to be prohibited under condition 3 of the PDE, we have seen that it is not the death of the foetus that is necessary for saving the woman's life; only the removal of the foetus is. If the foetus could be delivered alive, and kept alive, the mother might well avail herself of that option. And if she didn't, neither might the woman in Case *A*.

The point is this: if it is not the *removal* of the foetus that is prohibited by the PDE, but the *intentional termination of its life* (either as an end or as a means), then it is not clear how the latter is to be determined. Just as the fat man's death is not part of the potholer's plan, so the foetus's death need not be part of the woman's plan. In both cases, the agents could claim that their aims would not have been thwarted if the fat man or the foetus survived against all expectations. But if this is so, then the PDE would minimally sanction all those proportionate killings, where death itself is not an integral part of the agent's plan.

This is the view apparently accepted by one exponent of the PDE, Leonard Geddes. Geddes argues that, contrary to traditional Catholic teaching, a doctor who crushes the skull of a foetus in order to remove it from the womb and thus saves the mother's life is not

[23] Ibid.

intentionally killing the unborn child.[24] The foetus's death is itself neither an end at which the doctor aims, nor a means to some further end:

The surgeon must remove the child from the mother's womb; the dimensions of the child are such that if the surgeon attempts to remove it without changing these dimensions the mother will surely die. He therefore alters these dimensions in certain ways. A necessary but quite unneeded and unwanted consequence of this procedure is that the child dies. Clearly, the death of the child does not enter into consideration as a means to anything. So, in the relevant sense, the killing of the child was not intended by the surgeon, either as an end in itself or as a means to an end. Hence, it is a mistake to think that the principle concerning the killing of the innocent applies to [this] sort of killing . . .[25]

But if a deliberate craniotomy is not an instance of the intentional termination of life, what is? Provided the action in question can be redescribed in terms that do not make reference to the death, either as an end or as a means, an agent could intentionally decapitate another person, without such a decapitation being an instance of the intentional termination of life; the potholers could blow the fat man to pieces, without thereby being said to have intended his death, and Dudley and Stephens—adrift and foodless on a raft—could eat sparingly off the alive cabin boy, intending only to satisfy their hunger, not the cabin boy's foreseen death.[26]

Clearly, if Geddes's account is correct, it will reduce both the PDE and the absolute prohibitions it is meant to support to vacuity. R. A. Duff, intent on defending both absolutism and the PDE, is aware that Geddes's account generates 'sophistical and unacceptable conclusions'.[27] However, Duff's attempt to draw the distinction between the intentional and the non-intentional termination of life by way of the famous example of Captain Oates is hardly more successful than that of Geddes in limiting what the PDE allows.

[24] Traditional Catholic teaching prohibits the crushing of an unborn child's skull even in cases where *both* mother and child will die; see, for example, Holy Decree, May 1884. This ban was reiterated in the Holy Office Decree of 19 August 1889, and there widened to include a 'direct attack' upon the life of the foetus. (I owe these references to R. G. Frey: 'Some Aspects of the Doctrine of Double Effect', *Canadian Journal of Philosophy* 5 (1975), 268.)

[25] Leonard Geddes: 'On the Intrinsic Wrongness of Killing Innocent People', *Analysis* 33 (1973), 94–5.

[26] See *R. v. Dudley and Stephens* [1884] 14 QBD 273. For a discussion of the case, see R. A. Duff: 'Intentionally Killing the Innocent', *Analysis* 34 (1973), 16–19, and J. G. Hanink: 'Some Light on Double Effect', *Analysis* 35 (1975), 147–51.

[27] Duff: 'Absolute Principles and Double Effect', 68.

As Duff recounts the story, Oates 'walked out to certain death in a blizzard to give his friends a better chance of survival'. If Oates had shot himself, this would—according to Duff—have been an instance of the intentional termination of life and would have been ruled out by the absolute prohibition against intentionally taking life, either one's own or that of another. Merely to walk out, on the other hand is—Duff contends—not an instance of the intentional termination of life, even if 'death is equally certain in either case', and even if 'the end aimed at—of bringing his friends to go on without him which he knows they will not do while he is there with them—is the same'.[28] However, Duff contends, the

means adopted are crucially different. For in one case they will go on because he is dead and he intentionally kills himself, by shooting, as a means to this. But in the other case . . . he intends them to go on because they realize that he has chosen to withdraw from the group; and to achieve this, he needs simply to walk away.

Of course, he knows, and they know, that he will certainly die but this is now a consequence, not a part, of his intentional action. It is separable from it, in a way in which his death is not separable from shooting himself. This separation—this logical gap between what he intentionally does and his consequent death—is important, not because it allows him or them to hope that he will in fact survive (they had no such hope), but because it shows that his intention, and attention, need in no way be directed toward his death: the rest is up to God.[29]

As John Harris notes, Duff's account is not far removed from the sophistry of Geddes's:

Had Oates lacked the strength to remove himself from the group physically but possessed a revolver, he might have equally effectively disassociated himself by putting the barrel in his mouth, pulling the trigger and thinking 'whether or not I die is up to God'.[30]

It might seem that in the case of shooting himself, Oates has only succeeded in removing himself from the group if he does in fact die; in the case of walking away, he has removed himself whether or not he dies. But, then, Oates's aim, that the group go on without him, would not have been thwarted if the bullet had merely stunned him, so that his friends—thinking that it had killed him—would have walked on without him.

[28] Ibid., 78.
[29] Ibid., 78–9.
[30] Harris: *Violence and Responsibility*, 54.

Duff himself is aware that his account remains problematic, and cites a case where the problems inherent in the Captain Oates example are even more pronounced: A man throws himself on a live grenade to save his friends. This case is generally regarded as an instance of a man not intentionally destroying himself.[31] But if this man is said not to be killing himself intentionally, then, Duff admits, we cannot say what we would want to say—namely, that a person who throws another on a grenade is guilty of murder, or of intentionally killing him. Duff admits that he has no adequate answer as to how these problems might be resolved and, it appears, neither do other defenders of the PDE.[32]

To exclude such sophistical and self-defeating applications of the principle, defenders of the PDE might try to appeal to something like Philippa Foot's tentative criterion of 'closeness', whereby 'anything very close to what we are literally aiming at counts as if part of our aim';[33] or (alternatively) to limit the *logical* possibility of, say, someone surviving being blasted out of the opening of a cave to Philip Devine's requirement that the counter-factual scenario be 'non-fantastic'.[34] However, neither the criterion of closeness nor the requirement that imaginable counter-factual examples be non-fantastic can assist those who want to base a plausible account of intention on actual rulings given under the principle.

Philippa Foot holds that crushing an unborn child's skull and blowing a fat man out of a cave must be regarded as instances of the intentional termination of life because even if there were two events (skull-crushing and death; blowing to pieces and death), these would, according to Foot, be 'much too close for an application of the doctrine of double effect'.[35] Be this as it may, such a criterion of closeness cannot be employed by those who want to rely on the notion of intention underlying traditional rulings given under the PDE. Take the example of pyramid pain-killing. As we have seen, the Vatican's *Declaration on Euthanasia* sanctions the use of adequate amounts of pain-killing drugs, even if they bring about the patient's

---

[31] See, e.g., Devine: *The Ethics of Homicide*, 123.

[32] Duff: 'Absolute Principles and Double Effect', 79. See also Fried: *Right and Wrong*, 24; and John Finnis: 'The Rights and Wrongs of Abortion: A Reply to Judith Thomson', *Philosophy and Public Affairs* 2 (1973), 143–4. Finnis suggest that an answer as to when one should say that a bad effect is intended must, in many difficult cases, await judgement by 'the wise'.

[33] Foot: 'Abortion and Double Effect', 158.

[34] Devine: *The Ethics of Homicide*, 122–4.

[35] Foot: 'Abortion and Double Effect, 157–8.

death. Whilst the *Declaration* only speaks of a possible shortening of the patient's life, it is also recognized that it may be necessary to increase the dosage of pain-killing drugs in order to maintain their efficacy. It would seem, then, that in many cases the stage will be reached where a doctor foresees that a particular dosage which is sufficiently large to alleviate the patient's pain will also positively cause the patient's death. If Foot's criterion of 'closeness' were to determine what is or is not the intentional termination of life, then the doctor's action of deliberately administering what she believes to be a lethal dose of a pain-killing drug would clearly be an instance of the intentional termination of life.[36] And yet, according to traditional interpretations of the PDE, it is not: what the doctor is said to 'do' is merely to relieve the patient's pain. But, once again, if this is not an instance of the intentional termination of life, then it would seem, neither would be many other deliberate actions that defenders of the SLP would want to describe as such.

What about Devine's suggestion that a killing count as non-intentional (he calls it 'indirect') if there is some not too fantastic scenario according to which the action does not produce the lethal effect? This scenario, Devine says, 'need not be actually possible in the situation, [though it] must still not deviate too far from possibility and toward fantasy'.[37] But like Philippa Foot's criterion of 'closeness', Devine's criterion of empirical possibility cannot assist us in distinguishing between the intentional and the non-intentional termination of life. Not only would the notion of what an agent does intentionally depend, as Devine realizes, on such relative factors as the state of medical technology,[38] but this criterion would, again, allow more than those defending the distinction between intention and foresight would want to admit. It would, for example, allow both abortions *A* and *B*, since it is not a fantastic scenario to suppose that a foetus can survive a removal from the womb and be kept alive outside the womb, provided the *method* of abortion does not itself make such a scenario fantastic. Whilst Devine's criterion might thus rule out

---

[36] Philippa Foot does not explain what she means by 'closeness'. She is aware that someone who takes this line may 'have considerable difficulty in saying where the line is to be drawn' around what is 'too close' (ibid., 158). But this difficulty is only minor compared with the difficulty of explicating what is meant by 'too close' in this connection, and why 'closeness' (in what sense?) should have a bearing on the question of whether or not a foreseen effect is intended. (See also Sect. 3.3.)

[37] Devine: *The Ethics of Homicide*, 122–3.

[38] Ibid., 124.

such methods of abortion as vacuum aspiration and craniotomy that result in the physical destruction of the foetus, it would not rule out those abortions where the foetus is removed intact—something that could be ensured not only in Case *A* but presumably also in Case *B*.

In this connection, we might also recall condition 3 of the PDE. It defines a 'means' as an effect that is causally prior to the intended good effect:

The good effect must flow from the action at least as immediately (in order of causality, though not necessarily in the order of time) as the bad effect. In other words, the good effect must be produced directly by the action, not by the bad effect. Otherwise the agent would be using a bad means to a good end, which is never allowed.

This causality condition can, it seems, be met in at least all those situations where the foetus is removed intact from the woman's body. If a non-viable foetus is removed intact from the womb, the foetus's death will not be causally prior to its removal. Rather, death will occur upon or after its removal. But if this is so, then it is clear that the death of the foetus is not a causally necessary means to, say, relieving the woman's strained heart: the woman's heart is already relieved when the foetus is disconnected from her vascular system, and the foetus's death is thus a *side-effect* of what the doctor did intentionally: to relieve the woman's strained heart by disconnecting the foetus.

I conclude, therefore, that the foetus's *death* need not be a causally prior means to saving the woman's life, either in Case *A* or in Case *B*.

Similarly in the case of Tyrell's shooting William II: William II's death is not a causally necessary means for the achievement of Tyrrell's end of plundering the king. Not only might death have occurred *after* the plundering, but Tyrrell's aims would not have been thwarted had the king miraculously recovered after Tyrrell had completed his plundering. Thus even if two distinct human actions, such as killing and plundering, are involved, death need not be a causally necessary means for the achievement of the agent's end.[39]

What we are left with in the case of Abortions *A* and *B* is thus a prohibition to the effect that it is impermissible to 'directly' remove a foetus from a woman's body, but that it is permissible to 'indirectly' remove a foetus from her body when it is inside a cancerous womb whose removal is causally necessary to save the woman's life. This

---

[39] In this connection, Thomson's discussion: 'The Time of a Killing', 115–32, is of interest. If Tyrell shoots William II at $t_1$ and if, as a result, he dies at $t_2$, when did Tyrell kill the king (bring it about that the king is dead)? See also Ch. 2, n. 26.

distinction between 'direct' and 'indirect' death-producing actions is often part of the vocabulary of those who appeal to the Principle of Double Effect. I shall therefore discuss this distinction in the following section.

## 3.3 'DIRECT' AND 'INDIRECT' KILLINGS

### *3.31 Introduction*

The distinction between permissible and impermissible instances of bringing about the death of an innocent human being is often expressed in terms of the distinction between the 'direct' and the 'indirect' taking of human life.

'Direct' killings are those 'whose sole immediate effect is the death of a human being'; 'indirect' killings are those where 'death is the unavoidable accompaniment or result of a procedure which is immediately directed to the attainment of some other purpose, e.g., to the removal of a diseased organ'.[40] If we revert to Cases *A* and *B* discussed in Section 3.2, the life of the foetus in Case *A* is said to be taken 'indirectly', whereas the life of the foetus in Case *B* is said to be taken 'directly'. Furthermore, in the latter case it is, according to traditional Catholic teaching, irrelevant whether the foetus is killed within the womb, or whether the non-viable foetus is merely removed from the womb.[41]

What exactly the distinction between 'direct' and 'indirect' amounts to is not clear. I have seen no full exposition or defence of it anywhere in the philosophical literature, although it is frequently employed by those who appeal to the Principle of Double Effect. It is clear, though, that the direct/indirect distinction is generally used synonymously with the distinction between the intentional and the non-intentional termination of life. In addition to that, it seems to cover a range of factors (Jonathan Bennett calls them a 'jumble'),[42] such as brevity or absence of time lag between what the agent does with her hands and another person's death, spatial closeness, simplicity of causal connections, paucity of intervening physical objects, and so on. However, whilst these criteria of 'closeness' may often coincide with what supporters of the SLP want to regard as instances of the intentional termination of life, they do not always

---

[40] Kelly: *Medico-moral Problems*, 62.
[41] Ibid., 108; see also Devine: *The Ethics of Homicide*, 107.
[42] Bennett: 'Whatever the Consequences', 244, n. 5.

coincide. One example was already given in Section 3.2: the permissibility of pyramid pain-killing; another is, as we shall see, the permissibility of killing in self-defence.

### 3.32 Actions and Consequences

It is often thought that 'direct' killings are instances of the intentional termination of life because if a surgeon, say, crushes a foetus's head in order to remove it from the woman's body, or removes a non-viable foetus from the womb, she must intend killing the unborn child because the head-crushing or the removal *is* the killing.

At this point, a few remarks on an extremely complex topic must suffice. They will, however, I believe, be adequate for our purposes.

Killing is not a 'basic action', and if a medical procedure such as an abortion is at issue, it will always be possible to describe what the agent does in various ways. Put most simply, an agent's action could be described as 'removing a foetus', 'relieving a strained heart', 'saving a life', or 'killing a foetus'. This raises a question which has been implicit all along: where is the line between an action and its consequences to be drawn?[43] Whilst it may well be that the line can be drawn in various ways, let us see what the claim that the, say, head-crushing *is* the killing amounts to.[44]

The view that what I 'do' is identical with the causal consequences of the action seems to be supported by some action theories. G. E. M. Anscombe and Donald Davidson, for example, advance what Alvin Goldman calls the 'identity thesis'.[45] According to both Anscombe and Davidson, when John (1) moves his finger, (2) pulls the trigger, (3) fires the gun, and (4) kills Smith, he has not performed four distinct acts: all of these are one and the same act. On these views, John's moving his finger is identical with his killing Smith. Elizabeth Anscombe thus writes:

a single action can have many different descriptions, e.g., 'sawing a plank', 'sawing oak', 'sawing one of Smith's planks', making a squeaky noise with the saw', 'making a great deal of saw-dust', and so on and so on . . . Are we to say that the man who (intentionally) moves his arm, operates the pump,

[43] For two extreme views see, e.g., those of John Austin and J. J. C. Smart, as discussed in D'Arcy: *Human Acts*, 2–4.
[44] For such a position of 'harming' see Fried: *Right and Wrong*, 44. But see also Bennett: 'Morality and Consequences', vol. ii, p. 108.
[45] Alvin I. Goldman: *A Theory of Human Action* (Englewood Cliffs, NJ: Prentice Hall, 1970), 2.

replenishes the water supply, poisons the inhabitants, is performing *four* actions? Or only one? . . . In short, the only distinct action of his that is in question is this one, *A*. For moving his arm up and down with his fingers round the pump handle *is*, in these circumstances, operating the pump; and in these circumstances, it *is* replenishing the house water-supply; and, in these circumstances, it *is* poisoning the household. So there is one action with four descriptions . . .[46]

Similarly, Donald Davidson: 'I flip the switch, turn on the light, and illuminate the room. Unbeknownst to me I also alert a prowler to the fact that I am home. Here I do not do four things, but only one, of which four descriptions have been given.'[47] And, again: 'But what is the relation between my pointing the gun and pulling the trigger and my shooting the victim? The natural and, I think, correct answer is that the relation is that of identity.'[48]

This means that if an agent does *X* (kills the unborn child) by doing *Y* (crushing its head), then her *X*-ing is identical with her *Y*-ing; since the surgeon kills the child *by* crushing its head, it follows that the head-crushing is identical with the killing of the unborn child.

Whilst these views are plausible views of causal agency, they cannot be used to show that an agent intentionally brings about all the consequences of her action.

Davidson's example is a case in point: I intend to flip the switch, I intend to illuminate the room, but I do not intend to alert the prowler. Another example is, once again, the practice of pyramid pain-killing. Here a supporter of the SLP would want to say: the doctor intends to give the injection; she intends to kill the pain, but she does not intend to kill the patient.

What is evident from this is that the 'identity thesis' as stated needs to be complemented with a theory of intention if it is to be usefully employed in ethical theory: for example, and this is of course our present concern, does an agent intend all the foreseen consequences of her action? The answer to that question is supposedly supplied by the PDE and by the distinction drawn by some supporters of the sanctity-of-life view between 'direct' and 'indirect' killings.

[46] G. E. M. Anscombe: *Intention* (Oxford: Basil Blackwell, 1958), 11, 45, 46.

[47] Donald Davidson: 'Actions, Reasons and Causes', *The Journal of Philosophy* (1963), 686.

[48] Donald Davidson: 'The Logical Form of Action Sentences', in Nicholas Rescher (ed.): *The Logic of Decision and Action* (Pittsburgh: University of Pittsburgh Press, 1967), 84.

### 3.33   *The Causality Requirement*

How, then, are we to understand the distinction between the 'direct' and the 'indirect' termination of life? The literature is, as I have suggested, extremely vague on this. But the PDE's third condition stipulates what is required by way of causal 'simplicity' or 'closeness' between what the agent does and the intended good effect: 'the good effect must be produced directly by the action not by the bad effect. Otherwise the agent would be using a bad means to a good end.'

This, then, it would seem is the criterion of 'closeness' that is important to the intention/foresight distinction. It suggests that there are two kinds of causal structure. One kind is where the good end is achieved by way of a good or neutral means, with a foreseen but unwanted bad side-effect also flowing from the means; and one kind is where the good end is achieved by way of a bad means:[49]

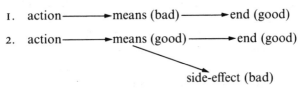

Thus, 'direct' intentional killings include those where death is a means to the agent's good end; 'indirect' unintended killings are those where death occurs as a side-effect of the means chosen to the agent's end. In the light of this causal structure, the distinction between the hysterectomy in Case *A* and the abortion performed on the woman suffering from a weak heart (Case *B*) thus derives its initial plausibility from the distinction between means and side-effects. The abortion of the foetus in Case *B* is regarded as a means to saving the woman's life, and is prohibited as an instance of 'direct' killing. The removal of the cancerous womb, on the other hand, is regarded as a permissible means to saving the woman's life, where the foreseen death of the foetus occurs as a side-effect of the means adopted to achieve the desired end.

We have already seen in Section 3.2 that the *death* of the foetus is not a causally necessary means to saving the woman's life in at least all those situations where the foetus is removed intact from the woman's womb. But let us assume that what a defender of the view that a difference in intention distinguishes Cases *A* and *B* has in mind

---

[49] This diagram owes much to Bennett: 'Morality and Consequences', 95.

is this: The agent who 'directly' removes the foetus from the woman's womb must, under the circumstances, intend its death, whereas the agent who removes the foetus only 'indirectly', that is, together with the womb, need not so intend because the hysterectomy in Case *A* would be performed *irrespective* of whether or not the cancerous womb contained a non-viable foetus. In Case *B*, on the other hand, it is precisely the presence of the foetus that threatens the woman's life: it is hence *its* removal that is causally necessary to saving the woman's life. Thus, whilst the foreseen death of the foetus need not be intended in Case *A*, it must be intended in Case *B*.

However, to draw the distinction between permissible and impermissible killings in this way will not help a supporter of this view, as killings that appear to be relevantly similar to Abortion *B* are permitted according to traditional interpretations of the sanctity-of-life doctrine: killings in the case of ectopic pregnancies and killings in self-defence. I begin by discussing the question of ectopic pregnancies.

*Ectopic pregnancies* Whilst traditional moral theology has not always permitted abortions in the case of ectopic pregnancies (because here the foetus's death was regarded as a means to saving the woman's life and therefore as an instance of 'direct' intentional killing),[50] it is now officially accepted that such abortions are permissible because the death of the foetus is brought about only 'indirectly', as a side-effect of what the agent does.[51]

This is surprising, because what Case *B* and the ectopic pregnancy have in common is that it is the presence and growth of the foetus that threatens the woman's life by, in Case *B*, overloading her weak heart and, in the case of an ectopic pregnancy, by causing a haemorrhage. When removing the foetus in either case, the doctor is thus not treating a pathological condition that is independent of the foetus's presence (as she does, for example, in Case *A*), but the foetus itself constitutes a threat to the woman's life. It is hence *its* removal that is causally necessary if the woman is to survive, and such removal would—according to traditional interpretations—constitute a direct

---

[50] Ruling of the 1900 Congress of the Holy Office, as cited by Joseph Fletcher: *Morals and Medicine* (Boston: Beacon Press, 1954), 150; see also Germain Grisez: *Abortion: The Myths, the Realities, and the Arguments* (New York: Corpus Books, 1970), 180.

[51] See, e.g., Bernard Häring: *Medical Ethics* (Notre Dame, Ind.: Fides Publ., 1973), 107; and Kelly: *Medico-moral Problems*, 105–10.

attack on the foetus. And yet, by ingenious arguments, of which Joseph B. McAllister's is a good example, it is now regarded as permissible to remove the foetus in the case of an ectopic pregnancy. A tubal pregnancy, McAllister explains, causes haemorrhage:

this can and should be stopped, not by attacking the foetus but by blocking the cause of the haemorrhage, by clamping the arteries. The foetus will die but as the indirect result of interrupting the blood supply to stop the haemorrhage. Then the tube and the dead foetus should be removed.[52]

Whilst one might be forgiven for thinking that an agent applying the Principle of Double Effect would have to postpone clamping the arteries until after the growing foetus has caused them to rupture, this is not the case. Rather, as Gerald Kelly, SJ, points out,

progress in medical research has shown that the tube itself is pathologically affected (e.g., because of the disintegration of the blood vessels, with consequent haemorrhage); hence, an operation to remove this condition is not a direct attack on the foetus, and is no longer condemned.[53]

It would appear, though, that even if it is accepted that the fallopian tube is in a pathological condition before it ruptures (and therefore somewhat similar to the cancerous uterus), it is difficult to maintain, on any plausible interpretation of what the agent intends, that to stop the vital blood supply to the cause of the pathology and the anticipated haemorrhage (the growing foetus!) is not relevantly similar to Abortion *B*, which is prohibited as a 'direct' attack on the foetus.

The point is this: if it is permissible to deprive the foetus, in the case of the ectopic pregnancy, of the necessary means for its survival (blood supply), why is it not also permissible to, for example, remove the intact foetus in Case *B* from the womb, thus depriving it of its means for survival (the womb)? To draw a distinction in this case is more than tenuous because it is, in both cases, the presence of the foetus that threatens the woman's life; and if it is permissible to bring about the foetus's death in one case by depriving it of its means for survival, it must be permissible to do so in the other. It cannot mark a distinction in the agent's intention that, in one case, she removes the foetus from the means necessary for its survival, and in the other,

---

[52] Joseph B. McAllister: *Ethics with Special Application to the Medical and Nursing Professions*, 2nd edn. (Philadelphia, 1955), 228, as cited by Glanville Williams: *The Sanctity of Life and the Criminal Law* (London: Faber & Faber, 1958), 202.

[53] Kelly: *Medico-moral Problems*, 109.

removes the means of survival from the foetus. Would the case be judged differently by a traditional moralist if, instead of aborting the foetus directly, the physician were to stop the blood supply to the placenta first, thus relieving the woman's pathologically affected heart of extra work, and then merely removing the placenta and the dead foetus? I think traditional moralists would have to say 'yes'. But if they did, it is not clear why they would judge this case differently. Just as the agent's end can now plausibly be described as 'relieving the woman's strained heart' (with the foetus's death now a merely foreseen consequence of the doctor's means, i.e. *clamping* the arteries), so the agent's end in Case *B* can be described as 'relieving the woman's strained heart' or 'correcting a pathological strain on her heart' (with the foetus's death now a merely foreseen consequence of what the doctor does as a means, i.e. *cutting* arteries). What is left, then, is the difference between clamping and cutting vital arteries. And why the agent who cuts the arteries is said to intend the foetus's death as a means, whereas the agent who clamps the arteries is not, I fail to see. Both agents intend to save the life of the woman, and initiate a causal process that they believe will inevitably result in the death of the foetus. If the death of the foetus is regarded as a means in one case, then so must it be in the other. Alternatively, if it is deemed permissible to bring about the death of a foetus in the case of an ectopic pregnancy by depriving it of its means for survival, then it must also be permissible to deprive other foetuses of their means of survival by removing them from the mother's womb in order to save her life.

I conclude, therefore, that the notion of what an agent 'directly intends as a means' does not allow us to distinguish between those abortions that are deemed permissible and those that are not.

*Self-defence and how impermissible means become permissible side-effects* I now want to suggest another reason why the notion of what an agent can be said to intend as a means will not carry the weight supporters of the SLP want to put on it. This reason lies in the *permissibility* of 'direct' killing in self-defence, and its close analogy (both in causal structure and in terms of what the agent can be said to intend) to other *prohibited* killings, including the abortion in Case *B*, and instances of euthanasia.

The justification of killing in self-defence goes back to Thomas

Aquinas,[54] and it is in his justification of such apparently 'direct' killings that the PDE is said to have had its origin.[55] Those writing in the tradition point out that agents may defend themselves not only against *unjust* aggression, but also against threats emanating from those who are morally innocent, including foetuses who threaten the life of the mother. If I am attacked by an insane person, I may kill the attacker—even though she could be incapable of moral responsibility and would hence be innocent in the required sense. If, in a case like that, I am permitted to do whatever is necessary to save my life, then it would seem that there will be instances where I may 'directly' kill another person. If a madman wields an axe at me and I can defend myself by shooting him in the leg, the second condition of the PDE stipulates that I do not aim at his heart. But if my only weapon is a stick of dynamite, then I am presumably permitted to throw it.[56] To be consistent with the SLP, this must either not be an instance of the intentional termination of life, or the person killed must not be innocent in the required sense. The first position is defended by Germain Grisez, the second by Alan Donagan. On both accounts, to be discussed below, abortions to save the mother's life are said to be permissible.

The questions of particular interest to us are these. How is 'direct' self-defensive killing justified in terms of the causal structure of the act and in terms of what the agent can be said to have intended; and how does this act differ, if it differs, from other instances of killing that are prohibited according to traditional interpretations of the sanctity-of-life doctrine?

For Thomas Aquinas, killing in self-defence is permissible because 'moral actions are characterized by what is intended, not by what falls outside the scope of intention'. It is instructive to quote him at length:

Nothing keeps one act from having two effects, one of which is in the scope of the agent's intention while the other falls outside that scope. Now moral actions are characterized by what is intended, not by what falls outside the scope of intention, for that is only incidental, as I explained previously.

Thus from the act of defending himself there can be two effects: self-preservation and the killing of the attacker. Therefore, this kind of act does

[54] Aquinas: *Summa Theologiae*, II, ii, question 64, article 7, response.

[55] See, e.g., Grisez: 'Toward a Consistent Natural Law Ethics'; another recent proponent of this view is Alan Donagan: *The Theory of Morality* (Chicago: University of Chicago Press 1977), 84–8.

[56] Uniacke: 'The Doctrine of Double Effect', 210–11.

not have the aspect of 'wrong' on the basis that one intends to save his own life, because it is only natural to everything to preserve itself in existence as best as it can. Still an action beginning from a good intention can become wrong if it is not proportionate to the end intended.

Consequently, if someone uses greater force than necessary to defend his own life, that will be wrong. But if he repels the attack with measured force, the defense will not be wrong. The law permits force to be repelled with measured force by one who is attacked without offering provocation. It is not necessary to salvation that a man forego this act of measured defense in order to avoid the killing of another, since each person is more strongly bound to safeguard his own life than that of another.

But since it is wrong to take human life except for the common good by public authority, as I already explained, it is wrong for a man to *intend* to kill another man in order to defend himself. The only exception is when a person having public authority intends in the line of duty to kill another in self-defence, as when a soldier fights the enemy or a lawman fights robbers. However, even these would sin if they acted out of private lust to kill.[57]

Central to Aquinas's argument for the permissibility of killing in self-defence are thus the notions of what the agent does as a means (defend himself) and what he intends as an end (preserve his life). Thus, as Grisez points out, Aquinas's argument is not 'that an intention to kill is justified, but that a performance of self-defensive behaviour which also kills can be intended as self-defensive and not as homicidal . . .'.[58]

The death of the attacker is thus neither an end, nor a means: it is a side-effect of what the agent does. This presupposes, as Grisez correctly realizes, that the act of self-defence, to be permissible, must be regarded as a unity, rather than as a number of different acts where, say, the agent's lethal stabbing is seen as a means to his end of self-defence. This view echoes the 'identity thesis' briefly discussed above. However, whereas on the identity thesis the act derived its unity from the causal process initiated by the agent, on Grisez's interpretation of Aquinas's view, an act derives its unity from two sources: the unity of the causal process, and the unity of the agent's intention.[59]

This means, Grisez says, that 'a good effect which in the order of nature is preceded in the performance by an evil effect need not be

[57] Aquinas: *Summa Theologiae*, II, ii.
[58] Grisez: 'Toward a Consistent Natural Law Ethics', 75.
[59] Ibid., 88–90.

regarded as a good end achieved by an evil means, provided the act is a unity and only the good is within the scope of intention'.[60]

In the light of our previous understanding of condition 3 of the PDE (Sect. 3.23, pp. 102–3), this interpretation does not appear to be saying anything new; here too the bad effect (the attacker's death) need not be causally prior to the good effect of saving the defender's life. What we may have overlooked, though, is that according to condition 2 of the PDE, an agent may not 'positively will' the bad effect. Is the agent's positively willing the impermissible, namely the 'direct' killing of an innocent human being, then *itself* such an evil 'effect'? It appears that it must be, because why else would the traditional moralist be at pains to drive a wedge between, for example, direct and indirect abortions, if—in either case—the *death* of the foetus need not be causally prior to the agent's good end of saving the woman's life? What appears to distinguish these cases on the traditional view, then, is that in cases of 'direct' killings it is held that the agent must positively *will* the bad effect before she moves her body in the appropriate way, and that this 'effect' (the forming of an intention) is necessarily causally prior to any further effects that we can observe *in* the world.

This, then, appears to be the view that Grisez challenges on the basis of the notion of intentional actions derived from Aquinas's justification of killing in self-defence: he holds that an agent need not 'positively will' the death of an innocent human being, even if life is taken 'directly'.

On this understanding of the PDE, Grisez says, 'Abraham would have been justified in sacrificing Isaac, since the very same act which killed Isaac would have been specified by Abraham's religious obedience as an act of worship'; 'a woman might interpose herself between her child and an attacking animal, since the unitary act would save the child as well as unintentionally damage the agent', but a woman 'could not commit adultery to obtain the release of her child, because the good effect would be through a distinct human act, and she would have to consent to the adulterous act as a means to the good end'.[61] As far as abortions to save the life of the mother are concerned, these would be permissible as unitary acts, provided the agent intended only the good effect (saving the woman's life) and not

[60] Ibid., 89–90.
[61] Grisez: 'Toward a Consistent Natural Law Ethics', 90.

the bad effect (the foetus's death). In other words, the moral nature of an indivisible act is determined by what the agent positively wills or intends as an 'interior act of the mind'.[62]

Perhaps this is also what Charles Fried has in mind when he says, in a previously cited quotation, that the intrinsic wrongness of killing lies in 'what it is wrong to do', where the principle's absolute force 'attaches only to what we intend and not to the whole range of things which come about as a result of what we do intentionally'.[63]

But, as it stands, Fried's definition of 'doing' is not very helpful. Do I intend all the foreseen effects that occur within a single causal process initiated by me, or is my 'willing' a unitary performance whose moral quality is determined by the intention '*with which*', to borrow from Elizabeth Anscombe, the act in each of its possible descriptions was done, and which 'so to speak swallows up all the preceding intentions *with* which earlier members of the series were done'?[64]

As we have seen, traditional interpretations of the PDE, which have gained explicit ecclesiastical approval in the Roman Catholic

[62] Elizabeth Anscombe is critical of this view, but does not put forward a consistent alternative account, other than to suggest that we must intend the means to our ends ('War and Murder', 51; *Intention*, 42). In *Intention*, 9, she says:

> Now it can easily seem that in general the question of what a man's intentions are is only authoritatively settled by him. One reason for this is that in general we are interested, not just in a man's intention *of* doing what he does, but in his intention *in* doing it, and this can very often not be seen from seeing what he does. Another is that in general the question whether he intends to do what he does just does not arise (because the answer is obvious); while if it does arise, it is rather often settled by asking him. And finally, a man can form an intention which he then does nothing to carry out, either because he is prevented or because he changes his mind: but the intention itself can be complete, although it remains a purely interior thing. All this conspires to make us think that if we want to know a man's intentions it is into the contents of his mind, and only into these, that we must enquire; and hence, that if we wish to understand what intention is, we must be investigating something whose existence is purely in the sphere of the mind; and that although intention issues in actions, and the way this happens also presents interesting questions, still what physically takes place, i.e., what a man actually does, is the very last thing we need consider in our enquiry. Whereas I wish to say that it is the first.

But if what a man actually 'does' is the first thing we need consider, it is not always—morally speaking—the most important. Because Anscombe grants that 'there will be cases where only a man himself can say whether he had a certain intention or not' (*Intention*, 44) and that an 'intention which is a purely interior matter nonetheless changes the whole character of things' (*Intention*, 48). It would follow, then, that whether an agent, say, 'defends himself' or 'kills the attacker' depends on just that: the interior act of willing one rather than the other.

[63] Fried, *Right and Wrong*, 20.
[64] Anscombe: *Intention*, 46.

Church during the last century or so,[65] hold that a bad or unwanted effect (death) of a 'direct' attack on life is intended not only when the good effect (unlike the bad) follows only in virtue of another human act (as in Grisez's example of the woman committing adultery to obtain the release of her child), but also when both the good effect and the bad effect are part of one natural process that requires no further causal intervention to achieve its aim. But is this view a defensible one?

My discussion in Section 3.2 showed that the agent need not intend the foetus's *death* as a causally necessary means to saving the woman's life in Case *B*. In this section, I want to go further: the notion of 'intended-as-a-means' is not a coherent one in the tradition we are discussing. The reason for this lies in the notion implicit in the PDE (as we shall see), that what an agent 'does' is determined not by what she brings about knowingly, voluntarily, and deliberately, but by what she intends as the end of her action.

For killing (the morally innocent) in self-defence to be permissible within the context of the absolute sanctity-of-life doctrine, the death of the aggressor must not be intended as a means to the agent's good end of saving her own life. This implies that the act of self-defence must be regarded as a unitary act, where the act is identical with all the consequences to which the doer's agency in performing it extends. The view that the agent's killing the agressor is one act and her self-defence another is untenable if 'direct' killing is, in this case, to be permissible: killing and self-defence must be seen as the same act, differently described. *How* the act is described depends on what the agent intends as her end. As Aquinas puts it: 'moral actions are characterized by what is intended and not by what falls outside the scope of intention'. Hence, the 'direct' killing of an aggressor, performed not with the intention of bringing about the aggressor's death but with the intention of preserving the agent's own life, is morally speaking not a killing but an act of self-defence. Self-defence is the means adopted by the agent to preserve her own life. Hence, from the moral point of view, killing in self-defence has not the causal structure previously shown under (1) on p. 106 above: rather, the line between action/means/consequences has been redrawn in the way it previously characterized 'indirect' killings as shown under (2). In other words, *where* the line between an action and its consequences

[65] John Finnis: 'The Rights and Wrongs of Abortion: A Reply to Judith Thomson', *Philosophy and Public Affairs* 2 (1973), 136.

falls is, in the tradition we are discussing, determined by what the agent intends as her end.

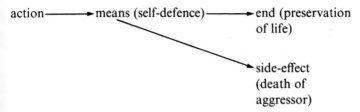

If the agent does not intend a death as her end, then she does not intend to kill as a means; rather, the 'means' to her end is self-defence, and this includes, if necessary, the killing of an innocent human being.

This, of course, is also the way in which Germain Grisez appears to understand Aquinas's justification of killing in self-defence and the Principle of Double Effect: that it is permissible to perform an intentional action which has two effects, one good and one bad, provided that the intention with which it is done is to bring about the good effect and not the bad. If this interpretation is correct, this would remove the difficulties the traditional moralist encounters in distinguishing, in terms of the agent's intention, between permissible and impermissible abortions. All abortions performed to save the life of the mother would be permissible because they would no longer constitute a 'direct' fatal attack on the foetus; the foetus's death would occur as a side-effect of what the agent does to save the woman's life. A corollary of this position and the sanctity-of-life doctrine (which does not distinguish between different types or kinds of human life) is that in cases where the doctor would be permitted to perform, say, a craniotomy to save the mother, she would 'be equally justified in cutting away the mother to rescue the baby'.[66]

Alan Donagan rejects Grisez's interpretation of the Thomistic principle of self-defence (and the PDE) and regards Grisez's conclusion—somewhat surprisingly, given his own framework of the equal inviolability of all human life—that the PDE would equally allow cutting away the mother, as 'shocking to the Hebrew–Christian tradition'.[67] Whilst Donagan, too, wants to allow abortions to save the mother, he argues that those abortions can be justified on the

[66] Grisez: 'Toward a Consistent Natural Law Ethics', 94.
[67] Donagan: *The Theory of Morality*, 162.

grounds that the foetus is an aggressor, whose life may be justly taken.

In taking this view Donagan is not alone, and his argument is representative of those of others who hold that it is never permissible to kill the innocent intentionally, and who also want to hold that capital punishment and killing in self-defence are permissible. This he attempts to do by arguing that those killed in self-defence and by capital punishment are not innocent.

The innocent, Donagan argues, are 'those [responsible agents] who are neither attacking other human beings nor have been condemned to death for a crime'.[68] On the basis of this definition of *moral* innocence (we are here concerned with 'responsible agents'), Donagan suggests that both capital punishment and killing in self-defence are permissible because the persons killed have lost their innocence and their protected status and may justifiably be killed to protect the lives of others.[69] I will not pursue this point. But what if the attacker is not a responsible agent? What if the attacker is an innocent foetus? To cover the mad person and the foetus, Donagan extends the notion of moral innocence to also cover *technical* innocence:[70] whilst the foetus who threatens the life of the mother is morally innocent, it is technically an aggressor, whose life may be taken, just as a beserk or drugged assailant may be killed if this is the only way in which an agent can save herself.[71]

Two comments on this: firstly, it is difficult to see how the permissibility of killing the *technically* guilty (but morally innocent) can be combined with the prohibitory rule against the intentional killing of the morally innocent;[72] secondly, if a person loses her protected status simply by virtue of being a non-intentional threat to another person's life, why cast the foetus and not the mother in the role of the aggressor? If the mother's pelvis, for example, poses a

[68] Ibid., 87.

[69] Ibid., 163.

[70] I have borrowed this notion of technical innocence from Judith Jarvis Thomson: 'Rights and Deaths', in Marshall Cohen *et al.* (eds.): *The Rights and Wrongs of Abortion* (Princeton: Princeton University Press, 1974), 122; see also Devine: *The Ethics of Homicide*, 152, where the author distinguishes between moral and causal innocence.

[71] Donagan: *The Theory of Morality*, 162.

[72] Based on the view that human life begins at conception, Pius XI and Paul VI, for example, hold that the prohibition of intentional killing applies to the *morally* innocent. On this view, the intentional killing of a foetus would always be wrong (because a foetus is always morally innocent), unless it can be justified by appeal to the PDE. See Sumner: *Abortion and Moral Theory*, 109.

threat to the foetus's life, why not remove the threat by cutting away the mother? Donagan regards this conclusion as 'shocking' because the foetus owes 'a debt of gratitude to its parents, and in particular to its mother, for its very life'. But this will not do to tilt the scales in favour of the mother. If the term 'innocence' is employed in its technical sense, lack of gratitude will not add anything to the argument; and if 'innocence' is employed in its moral sense, then, of course, the foetus is—as Donagan realizes—'utterly inculpable and innocent'. Perhaps realizing these difficulties and trying to limit what the argument from self-defence allows, Donagan admits a little later that 'what matters is not the innocence of the assailant but what is due to the victim'.[73] This may well be so; but if it is, then that is exactly the question the foetus, or someone arguing on its behalf, might want to raise.

I take it, then, that on either version of the argument from the permissibility of killing in self-defence, abortions to save the life of the mother, or instances of killing the mother to save the foetus, would be justified. An interesting question, not part of our present concern, remains: how does a supporter of these positions arrive at an acceptable, non-arbitrary principle as to whose life, that of the mother or the foetus, should be sacrificed in conflict situations where one but not both can live?

But also another question remains, and one that concerns us directly: in the light of the difficulties that the notion of the technically guilty (but morally innocent) raises for the Sanctity-of-Life Principle, will a supporter of the SLP grant that the permissibility of self-defence does not apply to the killing of the morally innocent, or accept (as, indeed, the original passage from Thomas Aquinas suggests) that killing in self-defence is based on the Principle of Double Effect? But if it is accepted that killing in self-defence is permissible, not because those killed are morally or technically guilty but because their deaths were not intended, then, of course, it follows that the notion of prohibited 'means' has no place in a single causal process initiated by a human act whose moral nature is determined by what the agent intends. Whilst it might initially seem more attractive to accept this narrow conception of the intentional according to which the moral nature of a unitary act is determined by what the agent intends, rather than to prohibit direct killing in self-defence— this option is not open to a defender of the SLP because both the PDE

[73] Donagan: *The Theory of Morality*, 162.

and the absolute prohibitions it is meant to support will be reduced to vacuity. There will no longer be any actions (such as the killing of the innocent, idolatry, sodomy, adultery, and so on) that are prohibited 'simply in virtue of their descriptions as such-and-such identifiable kinds of action':[74] an action would be impermissible only if the agent intended the impermissible as her end.

And yet, this is the position underlying not only Aquinas's justification of the permissibility of 'direct' killings in self-defence, but also that which is implicit in contemporary explications of the PDE. If an act is, morally speaking, the kind of act it is in virtue of what the agent intends as her mediate or ultimate end, then the notion of prohibited means becomes incomprehensible within a single human act—unless one holds the view that there is a certain class of acts that just *are* prohibited 'means', *irrespective* of what the agent intends as her end. But if this is the position underlying the Sanctity-of-Life Principle, then it would appear that the whole inquiry has got off on the wrong foot. What would be required is not the Principle of Double Effect, but rather a prohibition of voluntarily and deliberately bringing about the death of an innocent human being, or allowing such a death to occur, *irrespective* of what one intends as one's end.

Let me explain why this must be so. Conditions 2 and 3 of the PDE stipulate the requirements that must be fulfilled if the act is to be morally permissible. Take pyramid pain-killings, where the doctor, in order to relieve terminal pain, administers what she believes to be a lethal dose of morphine because a smaller dose of the drug would no longer alleviate the pain. Condition 2 of the PDE states that 'the agent must not positively will the bad effect'. Thus, if the doctor only intends to relieve pain (not to kill the patient), the act will, morally speaking, be good. In other words, the agent's end defines an act as good or bad in itself.

This act-defining character of the agent's intention is also important for condition 3, where it is stipulated that 'the good effect must flow from the action at least as immediately (in order of causality . . .) as the bad effect'. If the bad effect is causally prior to the good effect, it is suggested that the bad effect must be intended as a means, and it is impermissible to perform the act. But it is clear that this condition can always be fulfilled in the case of a single act whose moral nature is determined by condition 2: if the agent intends to relieve suffering,

[74] Anscombe: 'Modern Moral Philsophy', 10.

and if her 'means' is a lethal dose of morphine, then two effects will flow from this means: relief of suffering, and death. Since the agent intends only to relieve suffering and not the patient's death, she does not 'positively will' the bad effect; and in terms of causality, the prohibited effect (death) is not causally prior to the agent's end (the relief of suffering). Hence, the act is permissible, as will be all other proportionate acts whose moral nature is determined by what the agent intends as her 'good' end.

But this understanding of the PDE renders condition 1, that 'the act itself must be morally good or indifferent', strictly, superfluous:[75] an act can be good or bad only in virtue of *some* effect; and if an act is not permissible, then the performance of that act would involve the intention of what is bad, and this is prohibited by condition 2 of the PDE. Why, then, have the first condition? I suggest to rule out, in advance, certain acts that supporters of the Sanctity-of-Life Principle traditionally want to regard as impermissible, irrespective of what the agent can be said to have intended when performing the prohibited act: such as 'direct' abortions and the 'direct' killing of the innocent in general, idolatry, adultery, and so on. Whether or not an agent does, however, intend the death of a foetus whom she removes from the womb (or kills directly), is precisely the question at issue. It cannot be settled in advance. If 'direct' killing is permissible in the case of self-defence and in the case of pyramid pain-killing, it is permissible because, according to the PDE, the agent is said not to have intended the death in question. This is established by consulting conditions 2 and 3 of the PDE. But if this is so, then, of course, no 'direct' killings can be barred by condition 1, unless one accepts without further question that some acts, such as the direct removal of a non-viable foetus, just *are* instances of the intentional termination of life, whereas other acts that meet the same intentionality conditions just *are not*. However, I can see no reason for any such stipulative and apparently arbitrary classification and will consequently not examine that position.

## 3.34 Conclusion

I take it, then, that the PDE will permit all those killings where the death in question is not intended by the agent as her ultimate end. This has far-reaching implications, as a brief return to the question of

[75] See also Joseph M. Boyle, Jr.: 'Toward Understanding the Principle of Double Effect', *Ethics* 90 (1980), 532.

abortion will demonstrate. If an action of double effect is deemed permissible in virtue of (*a*) being a unitary act and (*b*) only the good being within the scope of the agent's intention, should not at least all therapeutic abortions be permissible under the same principle?

Here we must note an important distinction almost totally overlooked in the literature on the application of the PDE in the absolutist context: the distinction between the *permissibility* of an action in terms of the PDE's intentionality conditions, and the *justifiability* of an action in terms of the PDE's proportionality condition. This is something to which I shall return throughout the remainder of this chapter. Suffice it here to note that the two are not identical, and must not be conflated: an action is, according to the PDE, prima facie permissible if it meets the intentionality conditions (2 and 3); it is also justified if it meets the proportionality condition (4). That these two must not be conflated should be intuitively obvious from the fact that, say, saving the lives of five hundred at the expense of 'directly' killing one would be justified on the grounds of proportionality; it would, however, not be permissible if the one person's death would be directly intended. The question of central concern to us is the permissibility of an action in terms of the agent's intention: when can an agent be said to have intended a foreseen death?

On the present interpretation of the PDE, a woman would, for example, not be absolutely prohibited from having an abortion if the intent with which the abortion was performed was to forestall, say, the formation of varicose veins. If she were sincere in only intending the good effect (prevention of varicose veins), she would, according to the PDE, not intentionally be terminating the foetus's life. She might by *unjustified* in doing what she intends because the good effect may be deemed disproportionate to the bad effect according to condition 4 of the PDE. But if this is so, then the *reason* for the woman not being justified in doing what she intends lies in the substantive criteria of proportionality and not in the intentionality conditions of the PDE. Thus, if the action is morally permissible in terms of condition 2 of the PDE, and if there is a serious reason for undertaking it, then it may be done morally no matter what the foreseen consequence may be. As it stands, the woman may or may not be wrong in doing what she intends, but she would not be breaking the absolute rule against the intentional termination of life, and would not be doing what it is absolutely wrong to do: intentionally kill an innocent human being.

What is more—thus understood, a supporter of the Sanctity-of-Life Principle cannot appeal to the PDE to prohibit *any* proportionate 'direct' killings, where the death in question is not the agent's end. As already noted above, Abraham would have been permitted to directly kill Isaac, a 'soldier . . . can shoot straight at an enemy soldier, intending to lessen the enemy force by one gun, while not intending to kill', and a doctor could crush a baby stuck in the birth canal, or cut away the mother to free the baby, provided the doctor crushes 'no more than necessary to relieve the mother', and cuts no 'more than necessary to release the baby', because the excess damage, but not the necessary damage, 'would lie within the scope of intention and the act would be evil'.[76]

Now, many supporters of the SLP will want to reject the present interpretation of the PDE on the grounds that it permits far too much. Elizabeth Anscombe, herself a defender of the PDE and of absolute prohibitions, holds that whilst the denial of the PDE has been 'the corruption of non-Catholic thought', its abuse has been 'the corruption of Catholic thought'.[77] This abuse, she says, manifests itself *inter alia* in the alleged permissibility of obliteration bombing, where an agent is said to be permitted to bring about a large number of deaths, provided he 'secures by a "direction of intention" that any shedding of innocent human blood is "accidental" '; and in the somewhat quaint doctrine which says that *coitus reservatus* is permissible, whereas *coitus interruptus* is not: 'A man makes a practice of withdrawing, telling himself that he *intends* not to ejaculate; of course (if that is his practice), he usually does so, but then the event is "accidental" and *praeter intentionem*: it is, in short, a case of double effect.'[78]

One brief comment on the latter example: why is it thought to involve an 'abuse' of the PDE? If the man honestly intends not to ejaculate, then this would be sufficient to make his act an instance of *coitus reservatus*, irrespective of whether or not he ejaculates.[79] If acts were judged, by supporters of absolutist principles, by what an

[76] Grisez: 'Toward a Consistent Natural Law Ethics', 90, 91, 94.
[77] Anscombe: 'War and Murder', 46.
[78] Ibid., 51.
[79] See also Anscombe's comments on self-defence, ibid. Killing in self-defence is said to be permissible if the killing can 'in conscience' be said not to have been intended. If what the agent is said to have intended is sufficient to make the act one of self-defence rather than of killing, why is it not sufficient that the present agent 'in conscience' says that he intended not to ejaculate?

agent *foresees* will happen, then of course the gap between consequentialism and absolutism would have been closed—but this is not,
I trust, what Elizabeth Anscombe is aiming at, although I am not sure
how else her comments are to be understood.

What is clear, though, is that Elizabeth Anscombe, like other
supporters of absolutist principles, is acutely aware that absolutism
needs the PDE—she regards it as 'absolutely essential to Christian
ethics'.[80] She is also acutely aware that the PDE is being abused.
Unfortunately, we are not told *how* the PDE is to be understood and
how its abuse (if it is an abuse) can be prevented. Whilst Anscombe
makes reference to the notion of 'means' and suggests that 'direct'
killings involve impermissible means, she—like other defenders of the
SLP—fails to offer a consistent account of what constitutes either a
means or an instance of direct killing.[81]

Take killing in self-defence. This is permissible, Anscombe says,
under the conditions of the PDE, if the agent can in conscience say
'that the death of the other was not intended, but was a side-effect of
the measure taken to ward off the attack'.[82] 'Direct' killing in self-
defence would thus fall under the causal structure given under (2)
above (p. 106). Obliteration bombing, on the other hand, would be
characterized by the structure shown under (1) because in this case,
Anscombe holds, the civilian deaths are a means to the agent's chosen
end of (I suppose) defeating the enemy.[83] But if the bomber, like the
person killing in self-defence, were to say, in conscience, that the
foreseen deaths were not intended (the bomber would have avoided
them if the enemy could have been defeated in some other way), but
that they were a side-effect of the measures taken to defeat the enemy,
then I see no way of distinguishing between killing in self-defence and
obliteration bombing, either in terms of 'directness' or in terms of the
notion of 'means'. If anything, killing in self-defence would be more
'direct', in terms of the 'jumble of factors' of closeness mentioned at
the beginning of this section, than obliteration bombing would be.
There may, of course, be other ways of distinguishing morally
between the two cases, but whatever they may be, they would not
involve the notion of what the agent can be said to have intended as a
means.

[80] Anscombe: 'War and Murder', 50.
[81] Ibid., 51.
[82] Ibid., 45–6.
[83] Ibid., 51.

If the vague notions of 'direct'/'indirect' killings and 'intended as a means' do not allow us to distinguish between permissible and impermissible instances of bringing about an innocent human being's death, and if what the agent 'does' ultimately depends on what she intends as her end, then the PDE may not so much have been *abused* by Catholic moralists (as Elizabeth Anscombe thinks it has), but may merely have been interpreted in a plausible manner, especially given the claimed origin of the doctrine in Aquinas's views about self-defence.

What does emerge, though, is the following: if the distinction between the intentional and the non-intentional termination of life cannot be drawn in the way traditional moralists want it to be drawn, then it will be found that in all those cases where certain actions are not ruled out in advance 'simply in virtue of their description as such-and-such identifiable kinds of action',[84] the permissibility of the action will largely depend either on criteria of proportionality, or on other morally relevant factors, which are quite independent of the intention/foresight distinction.

It is to the showing of this that Chapter 4 is devoted, where I discuss the traditional distinction between 'ordinary' and 'extraordinary' means. First, however, we must determine whether the distinction between the intentional and the non-intentional termination of life cannot perhaps be drawn in some other way.

## 3.4   KILLING INTENTIONALLY AND REFRAINING FROM PREVENTING DEATH

### 3.41   Introduction

It is frequently thought that the killing/letting die distinction is morally significant because it marks a distinction in the agent's intention in relation to the death in question. Some writers in the field go so far as to claim that the killing/letting die distinction and the intention/foresight distinction are equivalent. Anglican moralists, for example, have implied that 'the distinction between rendering someone unconscious at the risk of killing him and killing him to render him unconscious' is the same as the distinction between 'allowing to die and killing'.[85] Similarly the philosopher R. A. Duff:

---

[84] Anscombe: 'Modern Moral Philosophy', 10.
[85] Anglican Church Information Office: *On Dying Well: An Anglican Contribution to the Debate on Euthanasia* (Church Information Office, 1979), 9.

in a previously cited quotation, he slides smoothly from the distinction between intending/foreseeing, over the distinction between acts and omissions, to the distinction between trying to harm someone and failing to avert harm, as if there had been no change of direction.

> We draw moral distinctions between what we intentionally do and what our actions foreseeably cause or what we fail to prevent; between the harm we intentionally cause and that which we fail to avert or which occurs as a by-product of some other intentional action; between trying to harm someone and recognizing that he will or may be injured by what we do: and we may sometimes allow the one while condemning the other.[86]

The passage conflates a number of issues, but this is not my present concern. My concern is to show that no plausible notion of intention seems to be available, which will allow us to distinguish—in terms of the agent's intention—between killing and letting die. Here we should remind ourselves that supporters of the SLP do not generally hold that letting die is never an instance of the intentional termination of life. Rather, they subscribe to the view—which is of course implicit in the qualified SLP—that ('direct') killings are always an instance of the intentional termination of life, whereas lettings die need not be.[87] This presupposes that a distinction in intention separates all killings from at least some instances of letting die.

### 3.42   Two Cases

Let us examine the distinction between killing and letting die by way of the following two examples. These examples are meant to isolate those features that might allow us to distinguish between instances of the intentional and the non-intentional termination of life. To achieve this, it is necessary that the cases be parallel in all relevant respects, except that one is a case of killing and the other a case of letting die. Only then can we be confident that we shall be able to isolate the difference in what the agent can be said to have intended.

1. Patient *C* is comatose and, as far as can be determined, will remain comatose until her death. She can be kept alive indefinitely with the assistance of a dialysis machine and an iron lung. The doctor believes that the patient would die within minutes if the iron lung were turned off.

[86] Duff: 'Absolute Principles and Double Effect', 74.
[87] See, e.g., Joseph M. Boyle, Jr.: 'On Killing and Letting Die', *New Scholasticism* 51 (1977), 434–5.

2. Patient *D* is also comatose and terminally ill. As far as can be determined, the patient will remain comatose until her death which will certainly occur within a few days. If she is given a certain amount of a drug by way of an intravenous injection, the doctor believes that the patient will die within a few minutes—just about the same length of time it would take Patient *C* to die if the iron lung were switched off.[88]

To make the cases relevantly similar, let us assume that the probabilities of death occurring as a consequence of the cessation of treatment in the case of Patient *C* and of administering the drug in the case of Patient *D* are the same (even though there is a difference as far as certainty of death *with* life-prolonging treatment is concerned: the death of Patient *D* would, under the circumstances, be more certain than the death of Patient *C*).

It is often thought that it is morally permissible to bring about the death of Patient *C* by discontinuing life-prolonging treatment, but not permissible to bring about the death of Patient *D* by administering a lethal injection, because the latter case is regarded as an instance of the intentional termination of life, whereas the former is not.

In this connection, we should recall the previous discussion of the PDE in determining whether or not it is, under certain circumstances, permissible to bring about a foetus's death. With regard to the intention/foresight distinction, Cases *C* and *D* are relevantly similar to Cases *A* and *B*. If treatment is discontinued in the case of Patient *C*, and the injection is administered in the case of Patient *D*, death—in either case—occurs as a consequence of an action of double effect, just as was the case with regard to foetuses *A* and *B*. Both actions have the good effect of, say, avoiding 'the investment of instruments and personnel . . . disproportionate to the results foreseen',[89] and the bad effect of bringing about the patient's death. What distinguishes *C* from *A*, *B*, and *D* is that death, in this case, is the result of a letting die, whereas death, in the other cases, occurs as a result of a killing.[90]

[88] These examples are based on two cases discussed by Gerard J. Hughes: 'Killing and Letting Die', *The Month*, 2nd NS (1975), 43–4.

[89] Sacred Congregation: *Declaration on Euthanasia*, 11. Under circumstances that meet this criterion, the *Declaration* deems it permissible to refrain from preventing death.

[90] There is one other difference, though, already mentioned above: we assumed that the deaths of foetuses *A* and *B* would be certain, regardless of whether or not the doctor performs the operation that will save the woman's life. The death of Patient *C*, on the other hand, is certain only if the doctor refrains from preventing her death.

Here we are primarily concerned with *C* and *D*, where the difference between them— the distinction between killing and letting die—should furnish us with a criterion as to how to distinguish between instances of the intentional and the non-intentional termination of life.

### 3.43   Means and Side-effects—Once More

On the by now familiar standard interpretation of the PDE, the two cases can be distinguished on the grounds that the death of Patient *C* is a side-effect of what the agent 'does', whereas the death of Patient *D* is a means to the agent's end. As one writer commenting on the case of Patient *D* puts it:

> The beneficent purposes which are often involved in euthanasia decisions cannot be realized unless the person is dead. Thus the pain and suffering and expense are ended only if the patient's life is terminated. The death, therefore, is a means of realizing these objectives and not a side-effect of their realization.[91]

Arguments rather similar to those already employed in arguing against the distinction in the abortion context can be advanced to show that the notion of 'intended as a means' will not help us to distinguish between the cases of Patients *C* and *D*. Since the argument is already familiar, I shall only state it briefly.

It is a mistake to assume that the doctor in Case *D* intends the *death* of his patient, whereas the doctor in Case *C* does not. Let us assume that the doctor in Case *D* administers what he takes to be a lethal injection and that, by some inexplicable process, the patient not only survives the injection but is cured by it. In this case, the doctor—just like Philippa Foot's driver of the runaway tram (Sect. 3.2), and the doctors in the abortion cases *A* and *B*—would not, we assume, ensure that the survivor dies some other way. On the contrary, one would expect him to be delighted to have achieved his objective, the avoidance of 'disproportionate medical treatment', without having had to bring about the patient's death. This shows that what the agent intends is not the patient's death but rather the avoidance of disproportionate treatment, with the patient's death being a foreseen side-effect of the doctor's action.

The point, to be discussed more fully in subsequent sections, is this: for treatment to be 'disproportionate' it must be disproportionate *to*

---

[91]   Boyle: 'On Killing and Letting Die', 436.

something. This 'something' is typically the patient's medical condition. (Ask yourself: would the doctor, other things being equal, turn off the iron lung if it sustained a patient not permanently comatose?) But if it is the patient's medical condition that makes treatment proportionate or disproportionate, then it is not the patient's *death* that is a causally necessary means for the achievement of the doctor's end (the avoidance of disproportionate treatment), rather it is the alleviation of the patient's medical condition. If this can be achieved in a way that does not entail the patient's death (for example, by curing the patient's medical condition), then the doctor would undoubtedly avail himself of this opportunity and not bring about the patient's death either by killing her or by letting her die. As things are, this alternative is not available, and the doctor can—without strictly intending the patient's death—bring about an avoidable death either by killing the patient or by letting her die.

So far it seems we cannot distinguish in terms of the agent's intentions between the doctor killing Patient *D* and the doctor letting Patient *C* die. Gerard J. Hughes, SJ—no radical—argues along similar lines when discussing these cases. He outlines the reasoning process the physician might go through when deliberating about the life or death of the patient in Case *C*. The physician might decide to terminate treatment because 'there is no point in doing anything further', and Hughes suggests:

he will come in for our moral criticism only if we discover that he also, for some disreputable reason, *wanted that patient dead*. The mere fact that the doctor performed an action—switching off a machine—will not in itself sway our judgment one way or the other, even though that action quite certainly results in the death of the person in a very short time.[92]

In the case of Patient *D*, the doctor could give 'a very parallel set of arguments' when he decides about the life or death of his patient, although it might be said at this point

that if he administers the injection it can only be because he intends the death of the patient. He would no doubt reply that it is certainly not true, any more than it was true in the case of the other doctor, that he *wanted the patient dead*. He had no ulterior motives, whether of eagerness to receive a legacy, or reluctance to see in front of him the continuing evidence of his own professional impotence to help. He did not in *that* sense want the patient dead.

[92] Hughes: 'Killing and Letting Die', 44.

It is true, Hughes grants, that

> he knowingly and deliberately did an action which had the death of his patient as an inevitable and immediate consequence. But then, so did the first doctor, and (yet) . . . the first doctor is allowed to say that he permitted the death but did not intend it.[93]

### 3.44   *Intending and Wanting Death*

Joseph M. Boyle attempts to defend the killing/letting die distinction against Hughes's attack. Since his defence is based on the intention/foresight distinction and is, to my knowledge, the most thorough discussion of that distinction in the present context, it will be instructive to examine his argument in some detail.

Boyle begins by arguing, against Hughes, that intentions and wants 'are not related in the simple manner which Hughes supposes'; rather

> When duty calls or necessity demands, a person will do and sometimes struggles to do what he does not want. Surely one intends to do what he does or strives to do. The sleepy workman does not want to get out of bed, but he intends to; he struggles and he does it. Generally, *someone's intending X* does not entail his wanting *X*. And *his not wanting X* is not inconsistent with *his intending X*.[94]

There is a sense of 'want' in which Boyle's claim is true. But if it is, it is not clear how the distinction between 'intending' and 'wanting', as Boyle draws it, will help us to distinguish between the cases of Patients *C* and *D*. The workman does not want to get out of bed for the sake of getting out of bed; but he knows that if he does not, he will (let us assume) lose his job. Hence, his getting out of bed is, in Bentham's terms, 'mediately intentional' (Sect. 3.23, p. 95). The workman has to choose between staying in bed and losing his job, or getting out of bed and keeping his job. *On balance*, the workman wants to keep his job; hence, *on balance*, the workman wants to get out of bed; he intends it and he does it. Similarly the doctors in Cases *C* and *D*. Neither doctor wants the patient's death for its own sake, but both want the patient's death more than the alternative: the continuation of what they see as futile treatment. So *on balance*, both doctors want the patient's death; they deliberate, and they do what they believe will result in their patient's death. So in *this* sense there is no distinction between what the doctors 'want' or 'intend'.

[93] Ibid.
[94] Boyle 'On Killing and Letting Die', 446 (emphases in original).

However, Boyle also suggests that there is 'some sense of "want" in which the second physician wants and the first does not want his respective patient's death'. Whilst neither physician is gleeful about the prospect of his patient's dying, and neither, we assume, stands to gain from his patient's death, the second physician nonetheless 'conditionally wanted his patient's death': 'Given his decision to kill the patient, the physician sets his mind on it. He acts to bring it about. If the first injection should fail, he would use another.'[95]

This decision to bring about his patient's death 'sets him on a course which, unless he changes his mind, leads to his patient's death'. It is in this sense of 'conditional want', Boyle argues, that the second physician is committed to his patient's death, whereas the first physician is not: 'the physician in the first case need not want the death of his patient in the conditional sense of "want". He does not try to bring it about. He need perform no action which presupposes a commitment to his patient's death.'[96]

But of course it is not true that the physician in Case *C* 'need not perform an action which presupposes a commitment to his patient's death'. If the physician decides to perform the action of turning off the iron lung *believing* that this will under the circumstances, bring about the patient's death, then he must also want the patient's death in some conditional sense of want. If he didn't, why would he deliberately and voluntarily do what he could refrain from doing? What is true is that the physician in Case *C* does not *kill* his patient, because he does not initiate a causal process that is, under the circumstances, sufficient to bring about the patient's death: he lets the patient die by refraining from preventing her death. But the distinction between killing and letting die is not co-extensive with the distinction between the intentional and the non-intentional termination of life, nor does it, as already shown in Chapter 2, coincide with the degree to which an agent is committed to, or wants, another person's death.

Boyle holds that in deciding to administer the lethal injection, the physician has set his mind on death: if the first injection should fail, he would administer another. This may well be true. But even if it is, it is not clear how this will allow us to distinguish between cases *C* and *D* on the basis of the agent's intention. When the physician in Case *C*

[95] Ibid.
[96] Ibid., 447.

decides to discontinue treatment, believing that this will bring about the patient's death, then he too must have 'set his mind on death'. To make the cases parallel, we assumed that both the doctor in Case *C* and the doctor in Case *D believe* that their respective patients will die if they do what they intend: administer an injection, or turn off an iron lung. Thus, at the level of intention, both doctors must—on balance—have wanted their patient's deaths. If, in the case of *C*, the patient totally unexpectedly survives, the doctor will not know this until after he has formed the intention to switch off the machine (believing then that this will inevitably result in the patient's death), and acted on it. Hence, there is no difference between the doctors on the level of what they can be said to have intended when they deliberately and voluntarily performed an action that they believed would result in their patient's death. If it is found that the belief of the doctor in Case *C* has been wrong, after the fact, this does not mean that he did not intend to do what this false belief entailed: bring about his patient's death. Hence, we cannot in *this* sense distinguish between the actions of the two doctors.

What, then, of Boyle's related point that, assuming the totally unexpected survival of both patients, the doctor in Case *D* would now administer a second injection, whereas the doctor in Case *C* would not ensure that his patient dies some other way?

Two comments on this: firstly, we have already seen that *even if* one, or both, patients survived, this would not show that there was a difference in what the agents intended when they acted the way they did, believing that their patients would die as a consequence of their actions; secondly, I grant that the doctor in Case *D* would, other things being equal, now administer a second injection. But is the situation substantially different in Case *C*? I think not. When a physician decides to discontinue 'disproportionate treatment' because, say, 'there is no point in doing anything further', and a patient, such as Patient *C*, inexplicably and totally unexpectedly survives without the iron lung in her comatose state, then—it would seem—the same reasoning that led to the decision to turn off the iron lung will logically lead to the physician now turning off the dialysis machine. The point is this: if the 'disproportionateness' or 'futility' of any further treatment is based on the patient's medical condition, then *any* medical treatment will, in certain cases, be disproportionate or futile as long as the patient's medical condition that prompted the judgement that 'there is no point in doing anything further' persists.[97]

Of course, if a patient not only survives but gets well when not treated, or when a machine such as an iron lung is turned off, then the doctor will not ensure that his patient dies some other way—but then neither would the doctor whose patient was cured by what he had believed to be a lethal injection. Thus, once again, killing and letting die cannot be distinguished in *this* sense of what each doctor can be said to intend when he kills his patient or when he lets his patient die.

It is sometimes suggested that there is another way of prying the two cases apart—namely, by appealing to the now widely accepted view of intention espoused by Elizabeth Anscombe in her book *Intention*.[98] If, as her analysis suggests, intentions are determined by the beliefs which motivate an agent's action, then it might be possible to establish a difference between the two doctors by asking how their behaviour would have differed if their beliefs had differed in certain ways. To this end, the following test question might be addressed to the two doctors:[99]

*If you had believed that your action would not have resulted in the patient's death, would you still have acted in the way you did?*

The answer to this question, one might initially expect, is that the doctor in Case *C* would answer 'yes' (because he would, even if his patient did not die, avoid the 'investment of instruments and personnel . . . disproportionate to the result foreseen') and the doctor in Case *D* 'no' (because there would be no saving of resources unless the patient were dead); and perhaps it is this counter-factual test Boyle has in mind when he suggests that the second physician 'conditionally' wants the patient's death, whereas the first doctor does not.

[97] Treatment may also be 'disproportionate' with regard to criteria other than the patient's medical condition—see Sect. 3.(53) and Ch. 4. For example, there may be cases where medical equipment is withdrawn from one patient because it is believed that it can more effectively be employed elsewhere, i.e., where the criterion of 'disproportionateness' relates not only to the patient's medical condition, but also to the relationship between a mean's employment in one case as against another. For example, a doctor may decide to withdraw the iron lung from Patient *C* to give it to Patient *Z*, who is not comatose. But even here the doctor who withdraws the iron lung from Patient *C* must, *on balance*, want his foreseen death: she would rather have Patient *C* than Patient *Z* die.

[99] The following discussion is inspired by Jonathan Bennett's analysis of the distinction between tactical and obliteration bombing in his Tanner Lectures on 'Morality and Consequences', 98–103.

We have already encountered the device of a counter-factual test in attempts to distinguish between permissible and impermissible abortions. However, whereas the counter-factual test could not help us to distinguish adequately between 'direct' and 'indirect' killings of a foetus, it would initially seem that the counter-factual test does indeed establish a difference in the doctors' intentions in Cases *C* and *D*. Whilst the doctor in Case *C* would presumably still have turned off the iron lung, even if he had believed that this would not result in the patient's death, it is implausible to suggest that the doctor in Case *D* would have administered the injection if he had believed that this would not bring about the patient's death.

But we must be careful in employing the test question to answer the question before us: whether a difference in intention distinguishes the actions of the doctors in Cases *C* and *D*. There are three ways of understanding the test question:

1. The doctor's state is to differ from his actual one *only* in respect of the belief that his patient would not die. This means that the doctor in Case *D* will still believe that his injection will result in the avoidance of the employment of 'instruments and personnel . . . disproportionate to the results foreseen', and the doctor in Case *C* has the same belief. In the light of this interpretation of the test question, both doctors would answer it in the affirmative: they would still have acted in the way they did. So this version of the test question does not separate the two doctors.

2. In the second version of the test question, the doctors' states are to differ from their actual ones in the belief that the patient would not die, together with whatever follows from that by virtue of all their other actual causal beliefs (which remain unchanged). Thus phrased, the doctor in Case *D* will answer 'no' to the test question: he would not have administered the lethal injection, for he supposes that there would be no death, and hence no saving of 'disproportionate means', because he has the causal belief that the resources can't be saved unless the patient is dead. But the doctor in Case *C* would also answer 'no' if asked the test question, because he too believes that there is no death, and hence he must believe there will be no saving of disproportionate resources (for he believes the resources are needed to keep the patient alive). So, again, this version of the

test question will not allow us to distinguish between the intentions of the two doctors.

3. But there is another way in which the doctors' states can differ. They can differ in so far as on this third reading of the test question, the doctors' supposed state is to differ from their actual one in the belief that their actions would not bring about the patients' deaths, together with whatever follows from that by virtue of what Jonathan Bennett calls a 'causally downstream inference'.[100] In other words, the adjustments are to be made with regard to what results and not with regard to what is causally pre-required. In the light of this reading, the doctor in Case *D* is supposed to be believing that there will be no death and therefore no savings in disproportionate resources; the doctor in Case *C*, on the other hand, is supposed to be believing that the patient will not die, but not that the machine will remain on—since the life-support machine is not causally downstream from the patient's death. In terms of this interpretation of the test question, the doctor in Case *D* will answer 'no' and the doctor in Case *C* will answer 'yes'. Thus, on this third reading, the doctor in Case *D* does and the doctor in Case *C* does not, intend the patient's death.

Whilst (3) is the usual reading of the test question, I believe that it is incorrect because it captures an illegitimately truncated notion of what the agent must, under the circumstances, believe if the cases are still to be relevantly similar. As we saw, the cases are parallel if the doctors' beliefs changed only in not including the belief that their respective patients would die, because in this case neither would refrain from his action; both would refrain from doing what they now intend if their beliefs would have changed in that way and in every way that causally follows from it. To pry them apart, it was necessary to stipulate that only what follows causally downstream (and not what is causally upstream) from the death in question would change. That assumption, I suggest, is illegitimate.

For the action in Case *C* to be one of letting die, or refraining from preventing death, it is necessary that a causal process not of the doctor's making already be in progress, which—together with the doctor's refraining—is sufficient to bring about the patient's death, and that the doctor be aware of this; if he were not aware of this, the

---

[100] Bennett: 'Morality and Consequences', 101.

doctor could not have the belief that his turning off the iron lung would result in the patient's death. Whilst the disease that led to Patient *C*'s being on the iron lung is thus causally upstream from the doctor's action of turning off the respirator, the doctor's action and what causally follows from it cannot be understood separately from what is causally upstream from it. It is only because of the patient's medical condition that the doctor's action is sufficient to bring about the patient's death. If we exclude beliefs about the causally upstream factors in the letting die case, we are leaving out what makes the doctor's action what it is: a letting die.

The test question—whether the doctor would still have acted in the way he did if he had believed that the patient's death would not have occurred—is thus misleading because it makes it easy to ignore causally upstream factors that are relevant to letting die but not to killing: whether, because of causally upstream factors, the agent's action or omission is under particular circumstances sufficient to bring about a patient's death. If it is, as it is in the case we are considering, then we cannot leave out the causally upstream factors that make the agent's action what it is: an instance of letting die, or of refraining from preventing death, rather than an instance of 'turning off an iron lung'. Hence, I suggest, the test question cannot be correctly understood in sense (3); and, of course, if it is read as either (1) or (2), there is no distinction between killing and letting die.

If this is correct, then either both doctors—or neither—'conditionally wanted' their patients' deaths. They would avoid the deaths if they could—that is, if they could achieve their aim (the saving of disproportionate resources) in some other way. But given the circumstances they find themselves in—that is, given the relevance of both causally upstream and causally downstream beliefs for the agent's understanding of their actions—they cannot turn off a machine necessary to keep a patient alive or administer a lethal injection if they do not intend their patients' deaths in the sense that Boyle gives to 'intend': that one intends to do what one does, on balance, want.

What distinguishes the two cases of Patients *C* and *D* is thus not a distinction in the agents' intentions: rather, it is the distinction between killing and letting die. In killing the agent initiates a causal process that is, under the circumstances, *causally downstream* sufficient to produce death; in letting die, the agent refrains from preventing death under circumstances where *causally upstream and causally downstream* factors are sufficient to produce death. To the extent that agents are, in particular circumstances, motivated by their beliefs about both causally upstream and causally downstream factors, I take it that there is no difference in the two doctors' intentions when they engage in, respectively, an act of killing or of letting die.

## 3.5     LETTING DIE

### *3.51     Introduction*

Supporters of the sanctity-of-life view generally believe that *all* instances of 'direct' killing, but *not all* instances of letting die, are instances of the intentional termination of life. This belief, captured in the qSLP allows the possibility that *some* cases of letting die are intentional. It is possible, then, that we were so far unable to isolate the difference between instances of the intentional and the non-intentional termination of life because the cases we have discussed were all cases in which a doctor brought about a preventable death intentionally. In other words, it might be that also the case of Patient *C* would be described by (some) supporters of the Sanctity-of-Life Principle as an instance of the intentional termination of life. It will therefore be necessary to look more closely at the distinction between what are taken to be instances of intentional and non-intentional lettings die to see whether we can discern a coherent and principled approach to this matter.

   Two claims are commonly made: that a difference in the medical conditions of patients, or in the means used to keep patients alive, will allow us to distinguish between those case where doctors brings about death intentionally and some other cases where death is merely a foreseen consequence of what the doctor does. I shall discuss these two claims in turn.

### *3.52     The 'Medical Condition' Argument*

It is sometimes claimed that we can distinguish between permissible lettings die by differentiating between different medical conditions. Joseph M. Boyle is an explicit exponent of this view,[101] but as we shall see in Chapter 4, many other writers in the field are implicitly

---

[101] Boyle: 'On Killing and Letting Die'.

relying on the patient's medical condition in their attempts to distinguish between permissible and impermissible lettings die.

Before we examine the question as to whether the distinction between the intentional and non-intentional termination of life can be supported by reference to the patient's medical condition, it is necessary to return to an important point, briefly touched on in Section 3.34: the differences between the *permissibility* of an action and its *justifiability*, and between the *intentionality conditions* and the *proportionality condition* of the Principle of Double Effect. Once these distinctions are drawn, it will, I believe, become clear that what is generally taken to be a conceptual and moral difference between intentional and non-intentional lettings die in the medical setting is typically a distinction between justified and unjustified lettings die. However, the question as to when we may justifiably let die is quite separate from the question as to whether or not we intend the death in question.

Let me explain. The Sanctity-of-Life Principle prohibits not the taking of innocent human life, or the bringing about of preventable deaths as such; rather, it proscribes that an agent *intentionally* bring about the deaths in question, either as an end or as a means, where the PDE's second and third conditions stipulate when an agent can be said to have intended the proscribed effect. These are *formal* requirements involving the distinction between means and ends and the further consequences of an agent's action. Moreover, since it is, on the view we are considering, always absolutely proscribed to intend the death of an innocent—*regardless* of the consequences— neither the good nor the bad effects, prudently to be weighed under condition 4 of the PDE, come into play when we are determining whether or not an act is absolutely prohibited on the basis of the intentionality conditions. Only when the intentionality conditions are satisfied will the proportionality condition come into play. As Germain Grisez, a supporter of the SLP, puts it: 'There is no point in discussing the justifiability of permitting the bad effects of an act which is admitted from the outset to be murder, quite apart from those effects.'[102]

It seems to follow quite clearly that the proscribed action, totally divorced from its consequences, consists in what Elizabeth Anscombe calls 'an interior act of the mind which [can] be produced at

---

[102] Grisez: 'Toward a Consistent Natural Law Ethics', 78.

will',[103] where this interior act of the mind is entirely independent of, and prior to, the consequences. Joseph M. Boyle gives a similar interpretation of the intentionality requirement. He holds that an action

> can be morally evaluated independently of either of its effects. Thus we may take the requirement that the agent intend only the good effect to refer to a human undertaking, the executing of a choice, which can be the subject of moral evaluation independent of the good and evil effects which are brought about.[104]

Whilst I will return to the notion of intention as an 'interior act of the mind' at a later stage, I think that it is sufficiently clear for our present purposes that the intentionality and the proportionality conditions of the PDE are quite distinct from each other, and that we are concerned, within the absolutist context of the SLP, with two questions, rather than one: (1) Is an action permissible in terms of what the agent is said to intend? and (2) If the action is not proscribed on account of what the agent intends, is it justifiable in the light of the proportionality condition?

What is self-evident, then, is that the question of whether an agent can be said to have intended a foreseen bad effect cannot be supported by criteria of proportionality, or by the claim that the agent is justified in acting as she intends by appealing to either consequentialist or other morally relevant considerations that are independent of the intentionality conditions. And yet, it is very often the case that the permissibility and justifiability of an action, or the intentionality and proportionality conditions of the PDE, are conflated in discussions involving absolute prohibitions. As an example of this, we might recall the example of a man throwing himself on a live grenade to save his friends. Commenting on the case, James Hanink suggests that even if it is not an 'intelligible human possibility' that the man survives, we would 'not want to say that he intentionally or wrongly killed himself'.[105] However, whether or not somebody intentionally kills himself is one thing; whether or not he also wrongly kills himself may be another. In his judgement that this is not an instance of the intentional termination of life, Hanink is in

---

[103] Anscombe: 'War and Murder', 51. Anscombe is critical of the view which regards intention as an interior act of the will, but she does not put forward a consistent alternative account. See n. 62.
[104] Boyle: 'Principle of Double Effects', 528; see also 531–2.
[105] Hanink: 'Some Light on Double Effect', 151.

agreement with traditional interpretors of the case, such as Philip Devine.[106] But if this is, on these views, not a case of intentional killing, why is it also traditionally held that a person who throws another on a live grenade is doing just that: intentionally and wrongly killing that person? What seems to be doing the work here is not the intentionality requirement of the PDE, but rather some notion to the effect that, say, voluntary self-sacrifice is morally acceptable, whereas the involuntary sacrifice of others is not.

Similar trends are apparent in the defence of the distinction between what are said to be intentional and non-intentional lettings die in the practice of medicine. Joseph M. Boyle's account is a case in point. Whilst the arguments I shall put forward are largely *ad hominem*, their implications are much wider than that. They can be directed against anyone who holds that we can, on the basis of the patient's medical condition, distinguish between the intentional and the non-intentional termination of life.

In his defence of the view that some cases of letting die are, and others are not, instances of the intentional termination of life, Boyle makes use of two cases. The first case, the famous Johns Hopkins case, is, according to Boyle, an instance of intentional letting die.

*Case E*   In this case a woman gave birth to a Down's syndrome baby at the Johns Hopkins Hospital in Baltimore, USA. The baby had an intestinal obstruction requiring routine surgery. If the operation is not performed, the child cannot take food and fluids orally and, unless fed intravenously, will die of dehydration and starvation. In this case, the parents did not consent to surgery and the baby was allowed to die.

In his discussion of this case, Boyle suggests that this was an instance of letting die 'which, in the opinion of many, was not justified'.[107] However, whilst letting die may or may not have been justified in this case, was it also an instance of the intentional termination of life? According to Boyle it was because, he says, the parents did not want to raise the child. In other words, 'the plan of action set forth by the parents involved the state of affairs of the child's being dead as an essential ingredient'.[108]

In suggesting that the death of Baby *E* involved the intentional

---

[106] Devine: *The Ethics of Homicide*, 123.
[107] Boyle: 'On Killing and Letting Die', 437.
[108] Ibid., 439.

termination of life, Boyle agrees with philosophers such as James Rachels.[109] However, whereas Rachels wants to suggest that *whenever* doctors refrain from preventing death they let die intentionally, Boyle argues that not all cases of refraining from preventing death are instances of the intentional termination of life. What distinguishes the Johns Hopkins case from other cases that are not instances of the intentional termination of life, Boyle argues, is the patient's medical condition and the nature of the treatment involved. Here I shall primarily discuss the claim that the distinction between the intentional and the non-intentional termination of life can be supported by reference to the patient's medical condition, leaving a fuller discussion of treatments or medical means to Section 3.53.

Referring to the Down's syndrome child, Boyle says:

> There seems to have been nothing wrong about the *medical* condition of the child's intestine or about the nature of the treatment which entered into [the] decision. In many cases of letting die, by contrast, it is precisely the patient's medical condition or the nature of the treatment which is relevant to the decision to let him die.[110]

Boyle then cites the following case where the patient's medical condition is relevant to the decision to withhold treatment and where, by extension, the patient's foreseen death is not intended.

*Case F*   A patient is dying of terminal cancer. The doctor withdraws life-support and, as a foreseen consequence, the patient dies.

In this case, Boyle suggests, treatment is withdrawn 'because of the relative futility or because of the pain it might cause, or the better use to which the facilities might be put'. Such reasons, Boyle argues, do not require that the doctor intend the death of the patient. Whilst the doctor foresees the patient's death and consents to it, 'he does not strive to bring it about. His aim is to avoid the use of expensive treatment and scarce facilities when their effects are foreseen to be marginal'.[111]

Whilst most of us would probably agree that there is an intuitive moral distinction between letting a salvageable mongoloid infant die by dehydration and starvation and not prolonging the life of a terminally ill and possibly suffering cancer patient, this different moral response does not have its locus in the intention/foresight

---

[109] Rachels: 'Active and Passive Euthanasia', 63–8.
[110] Boyle: 'On Killing and Letting Die', 438–9.
[111] Ibid., 439–40.

distinction. Rather, it would seem to lie in other morally relevant factors, such as the proportionate good that could have been achieved if the agent had not refrained from preventing death, quality-of-life considerations, and perhaps notions of justice.

However, considerations of proportionality or other morally relevant factors cannot supply the formal conditions that will allow a defender of the SLP to show that the agent in Case *E* did, and the agent in Case *F* did not, intend the patient's death.

If we accept that in Case *F* the agent's intention in letting die was to 'withhold relatively futile treatment that could be put to better use', then of course the agent in Case *E* might claim that she was similarly motivated. She might say that it is simply not the case that she wanted the infant dead. Rather, like the agent in Case *E*, she felt that here too treatment was 'relatively futile' and 'might be put to better use'. Of course, defenders of the intention/foresight distinction, like Joseph Boyle, might want to raise an objection here: they might want to say that treatment would not have been 'relatively futile' with regard to the Down's syndrome child. With treatment, they might say, the infant could have expected an almost normal life-span, whereas the cancer patient was expected to die shortly anyway. So the cases are, they could argue, substantially different.

But it is fairly clear that length of life is not in itself a relevant factor in determining intention: if I deliberately plunge a knife into the heart of a convicted criminal, scheduled to be hanged in a few hours' time, because I want to spare her what I believe to be a painful death, then I have terminated her life intentionally. It does not matter that had I refrained from doing as I intended, she would have died shortly anyway. Similarly with regard to letting die. If we imagine the convicted criminal as suffering from a temporary but severe bout of asthma which would be fatal were her breathing not sustained by an iron lung, then it would be possible for me to terminate her life just as effectively by switching off the iron lung as I could by stabbing her in the heart—and, again, I would have done so intentionally. Similarly in the medical setting: the fact that a patient is believed to be dying shortly anyway has no bearing on the question as to whether or not a doctor who refrains from preventing death has terminated life intentionally.

But perhaps we need to take a closer look at the patients' medical conditions. In Case *E*, Boyle suggests, treatment was refused not because of the patient's medical condition, nor because of the nature of the treatment involved, but rather because the infant was suffering from Down's syndrome. He suggests that the parents would have consented to the operation 'without hesitation if the baby were not a mongoloid'.[112] This may well be true, but if it is, then it is not obvious how this can help us to distinguish between Cases *E* and *F*. It is also reasonable to assume that the doctor in Case *F* would have employed life-prolonging treatment had the patient not suffered from cancer. Let us assume that the cancer patient, expected to die within a week, contracts pneumonia. This would, I believe, be a case where Boyle would want to say that it would be permissible for the doctor to refrain from preventing death by, say, not administering a life-saving injection of antibiotics because of the relative futility, and so on.

Of course, had the patient not suffered from cancer (other things being equal), then the doctor would unhesitatingly have administered the antibiotics and would not have refrained from preventing the patient's death. Seeing, however, that Patient *F* was suffering from cancer and that his underlying condition would be unaffected by the treatment, the doctor refrained from preventing his death. Whilst antibiotics would have prolonged the patient's life, such treatment would, just like the operation in Case *E*, have prolonged only a certain *kind* of life: life with terminal cancer and all its entailments in the one case, life with mongolism on the other. But if this is so, then Boyle cannot, on the basis of the patient's medical conditions and the nature of the treatments involved, distinguish between Cases *E* and *F*, or the intentional and the non-intentional termination of life.

Was death any more an essential ingredient in the agent's plans in Case *E* than it was in Case *F*? I think not. In either case, the agents could claim that they did not want the patient's *death*, that this was not what they were aiming at. All they wanted was to avoid treatment that would not cure the patient's underlying medical condition. If the cancer patient had miraculously shed his cancer, and the infant its mongolism, then neither agent would presumably have refrained from administering life-prolonging treatment. Since neither patient did, however, recover from the underlying condition that prompted the decision not to treat in the first place, both were allowed to die. Furthermore, since the decision to let die was voluntary and deliberate in either case, since the deaths were foreseen as inevitable or highly likely, and since neither agent (or both) wanted the patient

[112] Ibid.

dead, the two cases cannot be distinguished in terms of the intention/ foresight distinction. There may have been differences in the agent's motives: Boyle is probably correct when he suggests that the parents did not want to raise the child in its mongoloid state and thus acted from what some would regard as selfish motives; the doctor, on the other hand, seems to have been motivated by compassion when letting the cancer patient die. However, the distinction between different kinds of motives (whilst relevant to questions relating to the moral goodness or badness of *agents*, rather than the nature of their *actions*) is not in itself relevant for distinguishing between the intentional and the non-intentional termination of life. If I give someone a lethal injection, I may do so out of love or out of hate: 'to release a person from her awful suffering', or 'to no longer have to set eyes on the intolerable bastard'. Similarly with regard to letting die. If, as I think they would, defenders of the SLP would want to say that I have terminated life intentionally in either case, then the distinction between good and bad motives is not in itself relevant for determining intention.

This shows that distinctions in medical conditions and an agent's motivation in refraining from preventing death will not allow us to distinguish between instances of the intentional and non-intentional termination of life. This means that Boyle and those who think that it is the medical condition of the patient which is relevant to intention have but two consistent positions to choose from:

—to deny that in those cases refraining from preventing death is ever an instance of the intentional termination of life; or
—to accept that refraining from preventing death is always an instance of the intentional termination of life.

Both positions are rejected by supporters of the qualified SLP, who want to defend the view that some (but not all) instances of letting die are instances of the intentional termination of life. Whilst Boyle does not provide a satisfactory criterion as to how such a distinction could be drawn, a solution has traditionally been attempted in terms of the distinction between ordinary and extraordinary means of treatment.

### 3.53   *Ordinary and Extraordinary Means*

The distinction between 'ordinary' and 'extraordinary' means of treatment has a long history, especially in the Roman Catholic Church, where it was developed to deal with the problem of surgery prior to the development of antiseptics and anaesthesia. If a patient refused ordinary means—for example, food—such refusal was considered suicide, or the intentional termination of life. Refusal to use extraordinary means—for example, painful surgery—by the patient or the family, was not regarded as the intentional termination of life.[113]

I shall discuss the application of the ordinary/extraordinary means distinction within the sanctity-of-life doctrine in more detail in Chapter 4, where I shall argue that the distinction between so-called 'means' of treatment typically masks quality-of-life considerations, inadmissible as a principle for decision-making in the context of the SLP. Here I want to show briefly that the distinction between ordinary and extraordinary means is irrelevant to, and independent of, the question as to when an agent can be said to have terminated life intentionally.

The view than an agent who refrains from using extraordinary life-sustaining means is not intentionally terminating life is widespread. It is held not only by moral theologians[114] and by some philosophers[115] but is also implied by the much-discussed 1973 policy statement of the American Medical Association, which I quote in its entirety:

The intentional termination of the life of one human being by another—mercy killing—is contrary to that for which the medical profession stands and is contrary to the policy of the American Medical Association.

The cessation of the employment of extraordinary means to prolong the life of the body when there is irrefutable evidence that biological death is imminent is the decision of the patient and/or his immediate family. The advice and judgment of the physician should be freely available to the patient and/or his immediate family.[116]

Although issued by an American professional organization, this

[113] See T. L. Beauchamp and James F. Childress: *Principles of Biomedical Ethics* (New York: Oxford University Press, 1979), 117.

[114] See, e.g., Kelly: *Medico-moral Problems*; Sacred Congregation: *Declaration on Euthanasia*, 10–11; Chief Rabbi I. Jakobovits, as cited by Cardinal John Heenan: 'A Fascinating Story', 6.

[115] See, e.g., Bonnie Steinbock: 'The Intentional Termination of Life' in Steinbock (ed.): *Killing and Letting Die*, 69–77; see also my reply: 'Extraordinary Means and the Intentional Termination of Life', *Social Science and Medicine* 15F (1981), 117–21.

[116] Statement adopted by the House of Delegates of the American Medical Association on 3 December 1973. On 15 March 1986, the AMA issued a new policy statement. This statement still prohibits the intentional causation of death, while allowing the cessation of treatment, but it no longer makes reference to the distinction between ordinary and extraordinary means.

statement is not of exclusive relevance to the American scene. On the contrary, the attitudes expressed in it are accepted by physicians in many parts of the world.[117]

What, then, are extraordinary means of treatment? According to the standard definition:

Extraordinary means of preserving life . . . [are] all medicines, treatments and operations which cannot be obtained without excessive expense, pain or other inconvenience, or which, if used, would not offer a reasonable hope of benefit.

Ordinary treatment, on the other hand, comprises

all medicines, treatments, and operations, which offer a reasonable hope of benefit for the patient and which can be obtained and used without excessive expense, pain or other inconvenience.[118]

However, a long history does not guarantee clarity, and the Catholic Church has noted that even though the extraordinary means criterion 'as a principle still holds good', a reformulation is indicated 'by reason of the imprecision of the term and the rapid progress made in the treatment of sickness'. In the light of this, the Vatican's *Declaration on Euthanasia* continues,

some people prefer to speak of 'proportionate' or 'disproportionate' means. In any case, it will be possible to make a correct judgment as to the means by studying the type of treatment to be used, its degree of complexity or risk, its cost and the possibility of using it, and comparing these elements with the result that can be expected, taking into account the state of the sick person and his or her physical and moral resources.[119]

The distinction between ordinary and extraordinary, or proportionate and disproportionate, means of treatment is thus quite clearly an explication of the PDE's fourth condition, the proportionality criterion: whether an agent is required to prolong her own life or that of another depends on the proportion between the good and the bad effects that the treatment would produce.

We should note that the criteria explicated in the Vatican's *Declaration on Euthanasia*, such as probability, predictability, riskiness, cost, and so on, are highly morally significant. But we must also note that they are neither systematically connected with the

[117] See, e.g., Burton: *Medical Ethics and the Law*, 63; Singer, Kuhse, and Singer: 'The Treatment of Newborn Infants', 274–8.
[118] Kelly: *Medico-moral Problems*, 129.
[119] Sacred Congregation: *Declaration on Euthanasia*, 10.

distinction between ordinary and extraordinary means, nor with the distinction between the intentional and the non-intentional termination of life.

This is so for the following reason: a major factor in determining whether a means is optional (i.e., extraordinary or disproportionate), is the 'state of the sick person' and 'the result that can be expected'. A given means can thus be *either* ordinary *or* extraordinary, depending on the condition of the patient; the adjective 'optional' ('extraordinary' or 'disproportionate') refers not simply to the treatment considered on its own, but to the treatment in relation to the patient. In the case of the patient suffering from terminal cancer (Case *F*), for example, antibiotic treatment would, presumably, have been regarded as 'extraordinary' and hence optional. The same antibiotic treatment would, presumably, not be regarded as optional if an otherwise healthy person were to contract pneumonia. This point is explicitly made by one writer in the field, Bonnie Steinbock. What is 'extraordinary', she says, depends on the circumstances: 'The concept is flexible, and what might be considered "extraordinary" in one situation might be ordinary in another.' While the use of a respirator to sustain a patient through a severe but temporary ailment would be regarded as ordinary, its 'use to sustain the life of a severely brain-damaged person in an irreversible coma would be considered extraordinary'.[120]

Quite. But the criteria employed here are substantive criteria of justification that are independent of either the distinction between ordinary and extraordinary means (considered *as* means, or specific types of treatment) or the distinction between intentional and non-intentional lettings die. It may be that the agent would *not* have been justified in withholding an artificial respirator from a salvageable patient, and that she *was* justified in withholding a simple course of antibiotics from Patient *F*—and yet, considered independently from the patient's medical condition, a respirator is, on most plausible interpretations, more 'extraordinary' than a simple injection of antibiotics.[121] What is clear is that these justifications have little to do with means of treatment, and much with the quality and kind of life open to a particular patient with or after treatment.

Contrary to what is implied by the statement of the American Medical Association, the cessation of the employment of extraordi-

---

[120] Steinbock: 'The Intentional Termination of Life', 72.
[121] Kuhse and Singer: *Should the Baby Live?*, 30–7.

nary means *is* the intentional termination of life, based on the medical condition of the patient; and I conclude that the distinction between ordinary and extraordinary means can add nothing to the conclusion previously reached: either all lettings die are instances of the intentional termination of life, or none are.

### 3.6     THE PRINCIPLE OF DOUBLE EFFECT, ABSOLUTISM, AND RESPONSIBILITY

### 3.61     *Introduction: The Absolutist's Dilemma*

So far, we have been concerned with the manner in which supporters of the qualified SLP might attempt to distinguish between the intentional and the non-intentional termination of life. If my arguments have been correct, no plausible account of intention can be gleaned from actual rulings purportedly made on the basis of the PDE or the intention/foresight distinction: either all instances we discussed of an agent deliberately and voluntarily initiating a causal process or refraining from intervening in a causal process foreseen to lead to death are instances of the intentional termination of life, or none are.

The difficulty for supporters of the Sanctity-of-Life Principle arises from that principle's marriage to the PDE. This marriage is often seen not just as one of convenience, but as one of necessity. As the absolutist[122] Elizabeth Anscombe puts it:

If I am answerable for the foreseen consequences of an action or refusal, as much as for the action itself, then these [absolute] prohibitions break down. If someone innocent will die unless I do a wicked thing, then on this view I am his murderer in refusing: so all that is left to me is to weigh up evils. Here the theologian steps in with the principle of double effect and says: 'No, you are no murderer, if the man's death was neither your aim nor your chosen means, and if you had to act in the way that led to it or else do something absolutely forbidden.'[123]

But it is doubtful that the PDE can help the absolutist. As we have seen in Section 3.3, the notion of 'intended as a means' is an incoherent one if applied in the context of a single act whose moral nature is determined by what the agent intends as her mediate or

---

[122] The term 'absolutist' describes someone who believes that certain actions—such as the 'direct' killing of the innocent—are absolutely wrong in all circumstances, irrespective of the consequences.

[123] Anscombe: 'War and Murder', 50.

ultimate end. However, if this is so, then the difficulty for a supporter of the SLP arises at just this point: according to the PDE, an agent is permitted to bring about a proscribed effect intentionally (i.e. knowingly and deliberately), but is not permitted to directly intend (in the sense of 'desire', 'want', or 'aim at') the death in question. But if the SLP is based on this narrow conception of the intentional inherent in the PDE, then the SLP will become limitlessly permissive, ruling out the termination of life only in cases in which the agent desires the death for its own sake.

This is so because, as we have seen, what the agent 'does' is (according to the PDE) determined by what she intends as the end of her action. Hence, if the agent does not intend the death in question (but merely deliberately and knowingly brings it about), she does not terminate life intentionally. Rather, on this view, death will always be a side-effect of what the agent 'does'.

If my arguments in the preceding sections have been correct, this leaves supporters of the qualified SLP with but two choices:

—abandon the PDE and accept the broad conception of the intentional, according to which an agent terminates life intentionally *whenever* she could, by an act or omission, prevent a foreseen death and refrains from doing so; or

—retain the PDE and accept the narrow conception of the intentional, according to which an agent terminates life intentionally only when she intends the death in question as her end, or for its own sake.

Given these two choices, defenders of the qualified SLP face a dilemma. If they accept the broad conception of the intentional, their principle will be inconsistent because it would both prohibit and condone the intentional termination of life; while, if they accept the narrow conception of the intentional, their principle will be empty and no longer prohibit what supporters of the sanctity-of-life view have traditionally regarded as impermissible instances of the intentional termination of life.

What I have not shown, admittedly, is that there can be no 'intermediary' theory of the intentional which could, once developed, allow supporters of the qualified SLP to distinguish in a non-arbitrary way between instances of the intentional and non-intentional termination of life. I do not deny that there *could* be such a theory, but none has so far been presented; and until and unless such a theory has been developed, it would seem that supporters of the qualified SLP will have to choose between the broad and the narrow conception of the intentional. Moreover, as I shall argue towards the end of this section, even if such a theory were forthcoming, it would have to meet the charge of confusing the nature of *actions* with the moral dispositions of *agents*.

It might, however, be thought that there is yet another alternative: namely, to retain both the SLP and the PDE, and combine them with a thesis to the effect that there are certain actions, such as the 'direct' killing of the innocent, that are always wrong, irrespective of what an agent might have intended as the end of her action. This view is apparently taken by Elizabeth Anscombe when she suggests that there are certain kinds of action, such as murder or the deliberate killing of the innocent, where 'you do not have to think what you do is murder in order for it to be murder. What is necessary for your action to be murder is that you deliberately do such and such.'[124]

But if murder is thus what you 'do', irrespective of what you think or intend, why isn't the doctor who deliberately administers what she believes to be a lethal dose of morphine to her suffering patient doing just that: committing murder?[125] Or why isn't the doctor's refraining from preventing death (when she, for example, turns off an iron lung, does not administer antibiotics, does not operate, and so on) just that: the deliberate termination of innocent human lives, or murder? Conversely, why is it (as Anscombe suggests elsewhere) relevant to the permissibility of killing in self-defence that the agent can, in conscience, say that 'the death was not intended, but was a side-effect of the means taken to ward off the attack'?[126]

Philosophers, like other mortals, cannot have their cake and eat it: either what you intend as your end is relevant to the description of what you 'do', or it is not. Even if we accept with Eric D'Arcy, that there are certain acts of such moral significance that one cannot elide their description into terms which denote their further consequences, or into an end to which they were a means,[127] this will not help defenders of the SLP to separate what they want to regard as permissible and impermissible instances of bringing about a death, or of allowing a death to occur. We might, for example, agree that an

[124] G. E. M. Anscombe: 'Two Kinds of Error in Action', in Thomson and Dworkin (eds.): *Ethics*, 282.

[125] Elizabeth Anscombe thinks she does not: see 'War and Murder', 46.

[126] Ibid., 45.

[127] D'Arcy: *Human Acts*, 19.

avoidable death is always an event of great moral significance. But if it is, then it seems that it does not matter whether this death was brought about as a means or as a side-effect of what the agent 'did'. What matters is that the agent deliberately and voluntarily allowed a preventable death to occur, a death which is in either case a causally downstream consequence of the agent's action or omission. If this is correct, the absolutist's dilemma is still unresolved: it remains unclear how, and on what basis, the distinction between permissible and impermissible deaths is to be drawn.

### 3.62 *Doing Things Intentionally and Responsibility*

How might this dilemma be resolved? And when should we say that an agent has brought about a death intentionally? It seems to me that we should adopt the following position: to the extent that a death is the consequence of an agent's deliberate and voluntary decision, we should say that she brought it about intentionally—even if she did not intend it as her end, or for its own sake.

The terminology of intentionality suggests itself because of the close link between those things that we do intentionally and our responsibility for what we voluntarily and deliberately bring about. To distinguish those consequences that we intend as our ends from those that we bring about as side-effects of our intended actions, we might (with Bentham) distinguish between 'directly intentional' and 'obliquely intentional' consequences. Bentham draws this distinction in the following way:

A consequence may be said to be directly or lineally intentional, when the prospect of producing it constitutes one of the links in the chain of causes by which the person was determined to act. It may be said to be obliquely intentional when, although the consequence was in contemplation, and appeared likely to ensue in case of the act's being performed, yet the prospect of producing such a consequence did not constitute a link in the aforesaid chain.[128]

In drawing this distinction, Bentham is in agreement with other writers in the field,[129] including supporters of the SLP, although the terminology used is generally different. Supporters of the SLP usually restrict the terms 'intend' and 'intentional' to those consequences that an agent desires or wants to bring about as her mediate or ultimate

[128] Bentham: *Principles of Morals and Legislation*, 84.
[129] See, e.g., J. W. Meiland: *The Nature of Intention* (London: Methuen, 1970), 7–15; Meiland distinguishes between 'purposive' and 'non-purposive' intentions.

end. They then contrast these consequences with 'unintended' or 'unintentional' consequences that an agent does not want, but merely 'permits' or 'allows' to happen. Such terms can, however, be misleading. It is not only (as Stuart Hampshire and H. L. A. Hart point out), that the man who shoots someone knows, in a perfectly ordinary sense of 'knows', that his action will involve the production of a loud noise, and that it would hence be inappropriate to say that he made the noise 'unintentionally';[130] it is also that such terms as 'unintended' and 'unintentional' are ambiguous. To say that an agent did not intend $X$ can mean either that the agent brought $X$ about unintentionally in the sense in which it implies that she did not foresee it, or that she did not desire it as a means or as an end. R. A. Duff suggests that we could draw a stipulative distinction between *intending* a result and bringing about a result *intentionally*: 'An agent intends only those results whose expected or hoped for occurrence forms at least part of his reason for acting as he does; but brings about intentionally any result which informs his action, whether as a reason for the action or as a reason against.'[131]

Which terms we use is immaterial, as long as we use them consistently. To avoid ambiguity (and to point to the link between our responsibility for those things that we bring about deliberately and voluntarily, or intentionally), I shall employ Bentham's terms of 'oblique' and 'direct' intention. Moreover, I shall argue that—contrary to some recent views—lack of desire for a foreseen consequence is not, in itself, a factor that relieves a person of moral responsibility for the consequences of her voluntary and deliberate action. Indeed, this is the view underlying the PDE. The purpose of the PDE is not, as it is sometimes supposed, to absolve an agent of moral responsibility for the undesired consequences of her actions, but rather to give a ruling on the *permissibility* of an action, in terms of what the agent directly intends, and its *justifiability* in terms of both the directly and obliquely intentional consequences.

It is, however, frequently thought that the PDE is meant to give a ruling on an agent's responsibility for the consequences of her intentional doings: that we are either not, or at any rate somewhat less, responsible for the obliquely intended bad consequences of our actions. Elizabeth Anscombe, for example, regards as objectionable

---

[130] H. L. A. Hart and Stuart Hampshire are cited by D'Arcy: *Human Acts*, 171.

[131] R. A. Duff: 'Intention, Responsibility, and Double Effect', *The Philosophical Quarterly* 32 (1982), 3.

the view that 'it does not make any difference to a man's responsibility for something that he foresaw, that he felt no desire for it, either as an end or as a means'.[132] But why, it might be asked, should the fact that we do not desire a particular consequence diminish or abolish our responsibility for what we intentionally bring about? This question is raised by Henry Sidgwick, the target of Anscombe's attack. Sidgwick advocates the view that it is best, for the purposes of exact moral discussion,

to include under the term 'intention' all the consequences of an act that are foreseen as certain or probable; since it will be admitted that we cannot evade responsibility for any foreseen bad consequences of our acts by the plea that we felt no desire for them either for their own sake or as a means to ulterior ends: such undesired accompaniments of the desired results of our volitions are clearly chosen or willed by us.[133]

On Sidgwick's view, intention—and hence responsibility—thus extends to the directly and obliquely intended consequences of our actions, in so far as the latter are certain or highly probable. This position is formalized by Roderick Chisholm as follows:

If a rational man acts with the intention of bringing about a certain state of affairs $P$, and if he believes that by bringing about $P$, he will also bring about the conjunctive state of affairs $P$ and $Q$, then he does act with the intention of bringing about the conjunctive state of affairs $P$ and $Q$.[134]

How does this account of intention and responsibility compare with that inherent in the sanctity-of-life tradition? As we saw, no plausible account of intention can be extracted from actual rulings purportedly given under the PDE. In general, it would seem that intention (as used in the context of the PDE) implies 'want' or 'desire'; but a consequence can be foreseen and brought about without being wanted or desired. If what an agent does intentionally is equated with what she directly intends in the sense in which this implies that she desires it, it would follow that if one regards intention as necessary for responsibility, an agent is not responsible for the foreseen but undesired consequences of what she directly intends. Quite clearly, though, we are responsible for more than we directly intend.

[132] Anscombe: 'Modern Moral Philosophy', 11.
[133] Henry Sidgwick: *The Methods of Ethics*, 7th edn. (London: Macmillan, 1907), 202.
[134] Roderick M. Chisholm: 'The Structure of Intention', *The Journal of Philosophy* 67 (1970), 636.

It seems that the following connection between an agent's intentional action and her responsibility applies. When an agent acts intentionally, what she intends is that she bring about a certain consequence. She desires that consequence, either for its own sake or as a means to a further end. If the consequence of an agent's intended doing therefore occurs, she has brought it about intentionally. The term 'intentional' therefore denotes things done with the intention of doing them. But that an agent desires, or wants, a consequence is not necessary for having brought it about intentionally. Rather, what seems to be necessary for intentional action is the concept of deliberate and voluntary choice: if an agent *A* in doing what she intends believes that she will bring about not only *P* but also *Q*, and if she could have refrained from doing as she intends, then *A* has brought about *P* and *Q* intentionally because she has deliberately and voluntarily chosen to do what she could have refrained from doing. Since we are pre-eminently responsible for our intentional doings, *A* is responsible not only for *P* but also for *Q*.[135]

This presupposes that the agent has the *ability* and *opportunity* to refrain from doing as she intends, that she is *aware* of this and also of the fact that were she not to do what she intends, the consequence *Q* would not occur. When these conditions are met, *A* may not want or desire *Q*, but in voluntarily and deliberately choosing to do as she intends, she intentionally brings about not only *P* but also *Q*. And in thus acting intentionally, *A* is responsible for both *P* and *Q*.

To say this is, of course, not to deny that there will be situations where a person may be unable to voluntarily and deliberately choose a course of action because external constraints prevent her from doing so, or because her judgement is either temporarily or permanently impaired. Under circumstances such as these, an agent may be absolved of responsibility for the consequences of her deeds.[136] It is, however, obvious that the question of an agent being or not being responsible for the consequences of what she does must be kept separate from the issue of whether or not an agent is responsible for the bad consequences of her good actions *because she did not desire or want them*. Not being responsible for the consequences of one's actions because, say, one's judgement is impaired, is

---

[135] See George Graham: 'Doing Something Intentionally and Moral Responsibility', *Canadian Journal of Philosophy* 11 (1981), 667–77.

[136] However, here it should be noted that an agent is not absolved of responsibility simply in virtue of finding herself in a situation where she cannot choose deliberately and voluntarily. She would also have to show that she is not responsible for being in a situation where she can no longer exercise her choice.

one thing; not being responsible because one did not desire a consequence which one deliberately and voluntarily brought about is quite another.

Take the case of Patient *C* discussed above. Patient *C*, it will be remembered, is permanently comatose and can be kept alive indefinitely with the assistance of an iron lung and a dialysis machine. The physician assesses the situation and decides to turn off the iron lung because he wants to avoid the employment of what he regards as 'disproportionate treatment'. He does not desire the patient's death; he merely intends to discontinue what he regards as futile treatment, or too much effort for too little gain. The doctor knows that he can prevent the patient's death by refraining from doing as he intends (turning off the iron lung). But he does what he intends: he turns off the iron lung, which is an intentional action because it is intended. But in voluntarily and deliberately choosing to do as he intends, the doctor also intentionally brings about the patient's death, because it is a foreseen and avoidable outcome of his action. It is an inseparable part of a state of affairs which he brings about intentionally in preference to an alternative state of affairs which does not contain the patient's death.

As Sidgwick recognizes, in choosing to act as intended, an agent wills not only the intended result but also what she foresees as an inevitable or likely concomitant of her action. Although a doctor will often not desire to bring about her patients' deaths, she chooses to do so in all those situations where she *refrains* from preventing their deaths. Here we should remind ourselves that the relevant concept of choice is not that of choosing to perform a particular bodily movement—for no such movement need occur—rather, the concept is that for which choices are the issue of practical deliberation: and an action or omission was *chosen* when it was voluntary and deliberate.

In passing, we must note one objection: it is sometimes thought that an agent is not responsible for the bad consequences of her actions if she finds herself, through no fault of her own, in a situation where she must choose between necessary evils. A situation like this pertains in the case of the obstetrical example previously mentioned and in many other situations where the doctor must choose between, say, prolonging life and suffering, and bringing about the patient's death and thereby ending suffering. Take the obstetrical case. Here the doctor must choose between performing a craniotomy, thus killing the unborn child; or letting the mother die and delivering the child by post-mortem Caesarian section. Whilst most doctors would consider themselves bound to preserve and not to take life, it is implausible to suggest that the doctor who decides to let the mother die (because she believes that it is always wrong to perform a craniotomy, or because she believes that her role is, say, limited to preserving life by assisting certain natural processes) is not responsible for the foreseen but unwanted death of the mother—either because she did not want or desire the mother's death, or because she regarded it as 'unavoidable' in terms of her value system.[137] To see that role-perception as such does not absolve of responsibility, we need only to remind ourselves of those Nazi officials who claimed that they did not desire—and some of them positively disliked—the consequences they foresaw when they acted in accordance with their role or followed the dictates of duty. If we do not want to absolve them of responsibility for the undesired consequences of their actions, then we cannot absolve the doctor either: for it seems clear that the question of whether or not an agent is responsible for the foreseen undesired consequences of her actions does not depend on our moral judgements—it depends on her having brought them about deliberately and voluntarily.[138]

Similarly, the driver in our previous example of the runaway tram (Section 3.23): Whether he decides to stay on the present track, thus killing five, or decides to steer the tram onto the track occupied by one person, he is responsible for the consequences of what he intentionally does. Whilst it is true that in situations where an agent has to choose between unavoidable and undesired consequences, an element of compulsion or constraint is inherent in his choice, this does not mean that the agent is not responsible for the consequences of his choice within those constraints. Rather, what seems to be required in a situation such as this is a distinction between responsibility and blameworthiness—not in terms of the agent's intentions (he wants the death of neither the one nor the five), but in terms of the proportionality of avoidable and avoided consequences. If the agent steers the tram onto the track occupied by one person, he brings about the death of this person, and does so (within the constraints of the situation) deliberately and voluntarily. Whilst it is normally wrong deliberately to bring about the death of another person, it is—

---

[137] For a defence of the view I am attacking, see Casey: 'Actions and Consequences', 166–7.

[138] See also Frey: 'Doctrine of Double Effect', 259–83.

other things being equal—worse to bring about the death of five. Hence, the driver, whilst responsible for what he does, will not be blameworthy if he brings about one death rather than five. The constraints inherent in the situation do thus not absolve an agent of responsibility; rather, they provide excusing or justifying conditions for what it is normally wrong to do: deliberately to bring about the death of an innocent person.

The view sketched here, in affinity with that of Sidgwick, regarding the relationship between an agent's intentional actions and her responsibility for the foreseen bad consequences of her deeds, on the one hand, and her desire for those consequences either as a means or as an end, on the other, is not incompatible with either the PDE or traditional interpretations of the sanctity-of-life doctrine. Those writing in the tradition do not claim that an agent is not responsible for the bad consequences of her good actions. Rather, they regard a bad foreseen consequence as at least 'indirectly voluntary' and as such 'obliquely intentional', even if not intended or desired. An agent is thus traditionally deemed responsible for the foreseen bad consequences of her intentional doings. As Alan Donagan puts it:

In choosing to act according to a certain plan, a man thereby chooses to bring about *all* the causal consequences of doing so, whether or not they fall within his plan. He cannot escape responsibility by pleading that he did not desire or intend to do what he voluntarily did. And this is the traditional Hebrew–Christian position. The distinction drawn by some post-Reformation Roman Catholic Casuists between the directly and the indirectly voluntary, corresponding to what is intended as opposed to what is brought about voluntarily but unintentionally is therefore untenable. It is not drawn by Aquinas.[139]

To the extent that Elizabeth Anscombe claims to be writing in the Hebrew–Christian tradition, she is mistaken in thinking that lack of desire diminishes an agent's *responsibility* for the bad consequences of her deliberate and voluntary actions. Lack of desire for a consequence has a bearing, in this tradition, not on an agent's responsibility for the consequences of her action, but (for those who subscribe to the PDE) on the *permissibility* of an action.

This distinction between the moral permissibility of an action and

---

[139] Donagan: *The Theory of Morality*, 125. This point is also made by Boyle: 'Principle of Double Effect', 529–30, and by Gerard J. Hughes: 'Commentary: "Helga Kuhse: Extraordinary Means and the Sanctity of Life" ', *Journal of Medical Ethics* 7 (1981), 80.

the agent's responsibility for the bad consequences of what she does is most clearly drawn by Henry Keane in *A Primer of Moral Philosophy*:

In this type of action (i.e., inevitable evil consequence) a two-fold question arises:
1.   Am I responsible for an evil consequence which I foresee is bound to, or probably will, result from a good act of mine?
2.   Am I bound in view of such evil effect to refrain from the act in question?
The answer to (1) is sufficiently obvious. I am responsible. There is a causal relationship between my act and its consequences. As I am responsible for the act I am also responsible for that which directly follows from it.[140]

The purpose of the PDE, and the significance of establishing what the agent directly intends is thus, as Uniacke points out, to determine the answer to (2): Am I bound in view of such bad consequences to refrain from the act in question?[141] I am bound to refrain from the act in question if I intend or desire the bad consequence, but am permitted to bring it about as a secondary, obliquely intentional consequence of a good action. A case in point is the doctor who directly intends to relieve severe terminal pain by what she believes to be a lethal injection of morphine. If all conditions of the PDE are met, she may—as Hanink points out—*blamelessly* perform an action of double effect.[142] On the other hand, were the doctor, under the same circumstances, directly to intend the patient's death when administering the lethal dose of morphine, she would be to blame for having desired, aimed at, or wanted what it is impermissible to intend.

In this connection, we should recall the previously drawn distinction between the justifiability of an action in terms of the PDE's proportionality condition and the permissibility of an action in terms of the intentionality conditions. If an agent infringes the intentionality conditions, she is not *permitted* to perform the intended action: but even if she does not infringe the intentionality conditions, she may infringe the proportionality condition; and if she does, she is not *justified* in bringing about a death which she does not desire or intend. Blame is thus, in this tradition, apportioned on two accounts: when an agent intentionally brings about a disproportionate state of affairs, and when an agent intends what it is impermissible to intend.

---

[140] Henry Keane: *A Primer of Moral Philosophy*, Catholic Social Guild, Oxford (New York: P. J. Kenny & Sons, n.d.). I owe this reference to Uniacke: 'The Doctrine of Double Effect', 213.
[141] Uniacke: loc. cit.
[142] Hanink: 'Some Light on Double Effect', 150.

However, regardless of whether or not agents are also to *blame* for what they intentionally do, they are always responsible for the consequences of their intentional actions. When Elizabeth Anscombe rejects Sidgwick's above view of intentionality and responsibility on the grounds that it fails to take account of the difference in responsibility between desired and merely foreseen consequences, she equates the responsibility of agents for the *consequences* of their intentional actions with their blameworthiness for having *intended* what it is impermissible to intend. This becomes apparent when she suggests that a more appropriate account than the one proposed by Sidgwick is this: 'a man is responsible for the bad consequences of his bad actions, but gets no credit for the good ones, and contrariwise is not responsible for the bad consequences of his good actions . . .'.[143]

Here, it seems, Anscombe understands the man's being responsible for the consequences of his actions as the equivalent of being blameworthy for having infringed the intentionality conditions. But an agent's responsibility for the *consequences* of his deliberate and voluntary actions does not depend on the permissibility or impermissibility of his action in terms of the intentionality condition; rather, it depends on whether or not he has brought them about intentionally, that is, deliberately and voluntarily. I am responsible for all the consequences of my actions that I foresee as inevitably or highly likely because I *choose* to bring them about. Whether I am also to *blame* for what I have brought about depends on criteria of proportionality. For those who subscribe to the PDE or a related principle, I am also responsible for what I directly intend, and blame is apportioned if I intend what it is impermissible to intend: for example, the death of an innocent human being. This means that I am responsible for the directly and obliquely intended consequences of both good and bad actions, but that blame may be apportioned on two accounts:

1. that I directly intended the death of an innocent human being, even though I brought about a proportionate good;
2. that I brought about (without intending) the death of an innocent human being, and did not bring about a proportionate good.

Hence, what does distinguish the Hebrew–Christian tradition from the school of thought Anscombe is intent on attacking is not that for

---

[143] Anscombe: 'Modern Moral Philosophy', 12.

the latter foresight is proof of intention and hence of responsibility, but rather that for one strand of the Hebrew–Christian tradition (that strand which makes use of the PDE), an agent is deemed responsible for what she directly intends in addition to her responsibility for the consequences of her actions.

### 3.63   Actions and Agents

The question we need to examine next is this: what light, if any, does the notion that an agent is responsible not only for the consequences of her doings, but also for her *intentions*, throw on the permissibility or impermissibility of her actions and omissions? As we have repeatedly seen, according to the sanctity-of-life view, an agent who directly intends a death is not permitted to bring it about even if, did she not so intend, she would be permitted to bring the death about. To many an outsider to this tradition, the line drawn here seems very fine indeed. Glanville Williams, for example, scornfully rejects the distinction when he says:

It is altogether too artificial to say that a doctor who gives an overdose of a narcotic having in the forefront of his mind the aim of ending his patient's existence is guilty of sin, while the doctor who gives the same overdose in the same circumstances in order to relieve pain is not guilty of sin, provided he keeps his mind off the consequence which his professional training teaches him is inevitable, namely the death of his patient . . .[144]

Whilst I have great sympathy for Williams's sentiments, his introduction of the theological notion of 'sin' serves only to obscure matters. Specifically, it obscures the distinction between an agent's responsibility for the *consequences* of her intentional actions and her responsibility for what she *intends*, or desires. Both doctors are responsible for the consequences of their actions. The first doctor, however, is—in the context of the Catholic tradition and the PDE— also blameworthy for having directly intended what the other doctor only obliquely intended, the patient's death.

Thus, what seems to be the same thing can apparently be done differently by different people, with one person deemed blameworthy and the other not. The eleventh-century philosopher and theologian, Peter Abelard, gives a vivid illustration of this:

The same thing is often done by different people, justly by one and wickedly by another, as for example, if two men hang a criminal, one out of zeal for

[144] Williams: *Sanctity of Life and Criminal Law*, 286.

justice, and one out of hatred arising from an old enmity. Although it is the same action of hanging, and although they do indeed do what it is good to do and what justice requires, yet, through difference of intention, by the different men, the same thing is done by one badly, by the other well.[145]

This example is not without its ambiguities. I take it, however, that Abelard wants to suggest that one man acts rightly because he directly intends, or desires, to do what justice requires, whereas the other acts wrongly because he directly intends, or desires, the criminal's death. Whilst both men bring about the death intentionally, the first man directly intends it, whereas the other does not.

The notion that an agent is responsible both for what she directly intends in the sense of 'desires' and for the consequences of her intentional actions and omissions poses an obvious difficulty: it is permissible, according to the PDE, intentionally to bring about the foreseen death of a patient as a by-product of the alleviation of severe terminal pain, but it is impermissible to directly intend, or desire, the death in question. What if the doctor is simply not able to 'keep her mind off' the consequences of her action—if she intends not only to alleviate suffering but also the patient's death because she realizes that life is simply no longer of any value to the patient and believes that an early death would be in the patient's best interests? In this case, a doctor would be prohibited from doing what she would otherwise be permitted, and perhaps required, to do: alleviate pain with sufficiently large doses of drugs. But if a doctor both ought to alleviate pain and is not permitted to alleviate pain, then the theory that puts forward such opposing demands is seriously flawed.

If we now turn to Alan Donagan's 'solution' to this problem, we shall find encapsulated in it, quite neatly, the confusion that superficially holds the marriage of the PDE and the SLP together: the PDE's failure to distinguish between the goodness and badness of agents, and the rightness and wrongness of actions. Moreover, in the PDE's failure to draw this distinction lie the seeds of what Elizabeth Anscombe calls the PDE's 'abuse' in the Catholic tradition: that by a 'direction of intention', the impermissible becomes the permissible.[146]

---

[145] Peter Abelard: *Peter Aberlard's Ethics*, ed. and trans. D. E. Luscombe (Oxford: Clarendon Press, 1971), 28–9, as cited by Donagan: *The Theory of Morality*, 126.

[146] Anscombe: 'War and Morality', 51. Whilst Donagan rejects the PDE, he none the less supports the view I am attacking: that absolutely impermissible actions becomes permissible if the agents redirect their attention in the appropriate way. See Donagan, *The Theory of Morality*, 112–27.

Let us look, then, at the 'solution' advocated by Donagan. Donagan suggests that the problem of agents being both required and not permitted to do what their moral theory tells them to do can be overcome as follows:

Every rational agent has the power to determine his intentions. A man may have a motive to do wrong (as had Abelard's hangman, whose victim was an old enemy), but it is in his power not to intend to act on it. Abelard's hangman may, despite temptation, hang the criminal as his duty requires—namely humanely; and that intention will naturally show itself in various ways.[147]

Donagan suggests that a rational agent has the power to determine his intentions, and that even if he is motivated by, say, hatred rather than zeal for justice, the agent need not let the hatred colour his action: in hanging the criminal, he need not inflict more pain than is necessary. But that is *not* what Abelard—and indeed the PDE—suggests. Abelard holds that *even if* the agent performs the same kind of action (in terms of the humaneness of the hanging), one agent would be acting wrongly because he in some sense *wanted* the criminal's death, whereas the other agent did not. The agent who acts wrongly is motivated by the desire to bring about an old enemy's death. And to the extent that he wants the bad effect (the criminal's death), this agent is, according to Abelard, performing a bad action even if he hangs the criminal just as humanely as the other hangman does who acts out of zeal for justice.

This is, of course, the requirement that the agent must not 'positively will' the bad effect, as is stated in condition 2 of the PDE, and this requirement must be fulfilled *before* the agent initiates the causal chain of events in question because it determines whether the proposed action is prima facie permissible or not. But looked at it in this light, it will be obvious what condition 2 of the PDE amounts to: 'an interior act of the mind that can be produced at will'. Thus, what the hangman motivated by the desire to see his old enemy dead will have to do to make the hanging permissible is, as Anscombe ironically puts it in a related context, to address a little speech to himself to the effect that what he 'really wants' is to fulfil the demands

---

[147] Donagan: op. cit., 127.

of justice, pushing in the background of his mind the wish to see in front of him the lifeless body of his old enemy.[148]

Similarly the doctor in Glanville Williams's example: he must ensure that in the forefront of his mind is the thought that he will be relieving pain, rather than bringing about the patient's death, before his action becomes prima facie permissible.

However, whilst the PDE speaks about the moral nature of *actions*, what is at stake here is the question of *motivation* which is relevant to determining the moral dispositions of *agents*. Whilst a hangman who is motivated by the desire to inflict suffering may, other things being equal, be a worse kind of agent than a hangman motivated by zeal for justice, this does not mean that the agents perform different kinds of actions when they both hang the criminal humanely. Most importantly, it does not show that the first hangman kills intentionally whereas the second does not. I think supporters of the SLP will agree that both hangment intentionally terminate the criminal's life, one out of hatred, one out of zeal for justice. But if both hangmen terminate life intentionally, then the distinction between different motives or moral dispositions that give rise to the same action is irrelevant to the question of whether or not an agent terminated life intentionally.[149]

Of course, if a hangman's undesirable moral disposition 'show[s] itself in various ways' insofar as he might opt for an inhumane rather than a humane hanging, then the morally relevant difference between the two cases lies not in the intention/foresight distinction, but rather in the consequences of their actions: they do not bring about the same consequence (a humane death); rather, one brings about a humane and the other an inhumane death. Whilst both terminate life intentionally, one agent also intentionally inflicts harm over and above inflicting death.

Thus what gives superficial credibility to the marriage of the SLP and the PDE is the conflation of objective considerations concerning the rightness or wrongness of actions and the subjective considerations relevant to evaluating the moral character of the agent. If the

---

[148] Anscombe: 'War and Murder', 51; see also idem: *Intention*, 42–5.

[149] On the necessity to distinguish between (*a*) moral goodness, virtue and so on, and (*b*) the nature of actions, see William F. Frankena: 'McCormick and the Traditional Distinction', in Richard McCormick and Paul Ramsey (eds.): *Doing Evil to Achieve Good* (Chicago: Loyola University Press, 1978), 146–7. See also Boyle: 'Principle of Double Effect', 533.

SLP is meant to prohibit the intentional termination of life, it is irrelevant for that prohibition whether an agent acted from good or bad motives, or whether she desired death, either as a means or as an end; and yet, condition 2 of the PDE stipulates that the goodness or badness (and hence the prima facie permissibility) of an action is determined by what the agent intends, in the sense of 'desires' or 'wants'. This is where the confusion comes in: an agent must not, as we have seen, desire or want death, and yet may bring it about intentionally when she chooses to bring about a state of affairs *P*, believing that this will inevitably entail *Q*.

The difficulty I have pointed out here runs right through Elizabeth Anscombe's book *Intention*.[150] She suggests that intentional actions are those to which 'a certain sense of the question "why?" is given application'.[151] This question may be addressed to the man who (intentionally) moves his arm, operates the pump, replenishes the water supply and poisons the inhabitants.[152] 'Why are you moving your arm . . ., operating the pump . . ., replenishing the water supply . . ., poisoning the inhabitants?' If his answer is: 'To finish off the inhabitants', the case is unproblematic. But it is not if the operator were to answer: 'To earn my pay.'[153] Were he to give this answer rather than the first, he would not, on Anscombe's account, be poisoning the inhabitants intentionally: he would not be pumping *poisoned* water. Anscombe is aware of the problem and admits that 'we do seem to be in a bit of difficulty in finding the intentional act of poisoning those people, supposing that this (pumping water to earn his pay) is what his intentional act is'.[154]

Whilst there are, according to Anscombe, some checks as to what an acceptable answer to the 'why'-question can be, and whilst she holds that 'roughly speaking a man intends to do what he does',[155] Anscombe also admits that there are 'purely interior intentions' which, if meant, 'nevertheless [change] the whole character of things: . . . and make a difference to the correct account of the man's

---

[150] Anscombe: *Intention*.
[151] Ibid., 9.
[152] See Sect. 3.3.
[153] Anscombe: *Intention*, 40–1.
[154] Ibid., 42.
[155] Ibid., 43, 45.

action'.[156] But although *why* what a man does what he does may be of interest to our assessment of his character, it does not change the nature of his action. To the extent that a man voluntarily and deliberately brings about a bad effect, he brings it about intentionally and is responsible for what he does.[157]

## 3.64   Conclusion

With this, we have come full circle. If it is held that what an agent 'does' sometimes (Anscombe) or always (the PDE as we now understand it) depends on what she intends as her end by way of an interior act of the mind, rather than on what she voluntarily and deliberately brings about, then such a position fails to distinguish between the nature of actions and the character or motivations of agents. Moreover, it cannot be invoked by supporters of the SLP because it would allow far too much, ruling out the termination of life only in those circumstances where the agent allowed death to be in the forefront of her mind.

In the absence of a plausible intermediary theory of the intentional, this leaves supporters of the SLP with the other alternative sketched at the beginning of this section; to accept that an agent terminates life intentionally whenever she voluntarily and deliberately brings about a death or refrains from preventing a death. But if supporters of the SLP were to accept this alternative, their principle would become

---

[156] Ibid., 48. In this connection the Linacre Centre Working Party Report on *Euthanasia and Clinical Practice: Trends, Principles and Alternatives* (London: Linacre Centre, 1982), 48–9 is of interest—not least because Elizabeth Anscombe was a member of this working party. Under an item 'Refusing Treatment, Suicide and the Direction of the Will: Further Analysis', the working party concludes that whilst it is wrong to omit treatment because one judges life to be no longer worthwhile, it may nevertheless be permissible to refuse treatment, provided one ensures by a 'direction of the will' that one does not aim at death; rather the patient should attempt to see his refusal of life-prolonging treatment in terms of the non-obligatory nature of treatment. The report acknowledges that there must be some difficulty in practice over distinguishing these decisions which 'might appear identical', but, it continues, what matters morally are the patient's intentions and dispositions: 'The non-public character of the distinction . . . does not make the distinction unreal or less than fundamental.'

[157] Anscombe seems to agree: about the man who knowingly poisons the household but describes his objective as 'wanting to earn his pay', she says: his intention is 'certainly not of ethical or legal interest; if what he said was true, *that* will not absolve him from guilt of murder'. And, she continues, 'we just *are* interested in what is true about the man in this kind of way' because it tells us something about him which goes beyond what happened at the time (Anscombe: *Intention*, 45).

untenable: for it might require them to kill one innocent person to save the lives of five.

As will be recalled, the difficulty for the SLP arises because the notion of 'intended-as-a-means' cannot bear the weight exponents of the PDE want to put on it. Not only is the concept inconsistently applied by those who use it as a load-bearing part of their morality, but the whole notion becomes vacuous when applied in the context of an action whose moral nature is said to be determined by what the agent intends as her end. If the agent does not intend the death in question as her end, then she does not intend to kill or let die as a means. Rather, the death in question will always be a side-effect of what the agent does—for example, removing a foetus from a woman's womb in order to save her life.

As I said at the beginning of this section, I have not shown that there could not be an 'intermediary' theory of the intentional which might, once analysed, allow supporters of the SLP to distinguish in a consistent and non-arbitrary way between what they want to regard as instances of the intentional and non-intentional termination of life. But by having shown (conclusively, I think) that the judgements of those who subscribe to the SLP lack both consistency and a conceptually sound basis, I believe that the onus of proof is now on those who want to continue to subscribe to the sanctity-of-life view. In other words, I think I am justified in claiming that the SLP is inconsistent—until I have been proved wrong.

But let us consider what options are open to supporters of the SLP in the absence of such an 'intermediary' theory of the intentional. It might be thought that we can settle the question of permissible/ impermissible means on a case-by-case basis in all those situations where the chosen means will inevitably or very probably involve a foreseen death. As Elizabeth Anscombe says, there will be twilight, 'but the fact of twilight does not mean that you cannot tell day from night'.[158]

Thus it might be thought that we can settle questions as to what an agent can be said to have intended as a means and what were the side-effects of what she did on a case-by-case basis—confident that we might achieve consensus in the cases that are intuitively clear, prepared to arbitrate in the case of those that are not. However, I do not regard this as an acceptable approach to ethics. Ethics needs to be

---

[158] Anscombe: 'War and Murder', 52.

more firmly grounded in the nature of things, rather than in the intuitive or linguistic judgements of individual moral agents.

One such grounding can be found in the notion of causation (discussed in Ch. 2), which shows that agents, by their actions and refrainings, bring about certain consequences in the world. Another is in the notion of intention: moral agents do not just bring about certain consequences in the world, they bring them about intentionally and are responsible for them because they have brought them about voluntarily and deliberately. Looked at in this light, the distinction between 'intended-as-a-means' and 'foreseen as a side-effect' becomes immaterial (if it had not already been disposed of). What matters is not whether an agent brings about a foreseen consequence as a means or as a side-effect of what she 'does', but rather that she freely chooses to bring about a state of affairs that includes the said consequence, in preference to another state of affairs which does not.

To conclude, then, I believe that the Sanctity-of-Life Principle is untenable: if supporters of the SLP accept the broad conception of the intentional as outlined by me, the demands of their principle cannot be met—neither by complete inactivity nor by frantic activity. Whatever they choose to do, there will be situations where they would be breaking the absolute prohibition against the intentional termination of life. Moreover, in holding that it is sometimes permissible to allow a patient to die, the qualified SLP is inconsistent—for it both prohibits and permits the intentional termination of life.

In the next chapter, Chapter 4, I shall be dealing with yet another inconsistency which is often implicit in the life and death judgements of those who subscribe to the sanctity-of-life view. The SLP excludes the use of quality-of-life considerations; yet I shall show that the life and death judgements of supporters of the sanctity-of-life view are typically based on just such considerations.

# 4

# Extraordinary Lives—Not Extraordinary Means

... The language of ordinary and extraordinary means ... is ... an honored and useful distinction in Catholic moral theology as it applies to medical care. The principle is that a physician is under no obligation to use extraordinary means to sustain life. The difficulty in the application of the principle is the choice of what falls under extraordinary means. Under one set of circumstances a procedure may be judged ordinary, and under another extraordinary.

> James M. Gustafson: 'Mongolism and the Right to Life', *Perspectives in Biology and Medicine*, 1973

It is not necessary to be troubled by ambiguities attaching to the terms 'ordinary' or 'extraordinary'. It is the underlying considerations determining when treatment is obligatory which are important.

> *Euthanasia and Clinical Practice—The Report of a Working Party*, The Linacre Centre, 1982

Squirm as we may to avoid the inevitable, it seems time to admit to ourselves that there is simply no hiding place and that we must shoulder the responsibility of deciding to act in such a way as to hasten the declining trajectories of some lives, while doing our best to slow down the decline of others. And we have to do this on the basis of some judgement on the quality of lives in question.

> R. S. Morison: 'Death: Process or Event?', *Science*, 1971

## 4.1 INTRODUCTION

If my arguments in the preceding chapters have been correct, the qualified Sanctity-of-Life Principle is untenable because it both prohibits and condones the intentional termination of life. With this I could have concluded my critique of the Sanctity-of-Life Doctrine in the practice of medicine—for it would seem that after a charge as serious as this, any additional criticism is superfluous.

There is, however, another issue well worth scrutinizing: the distinction between so-called 'ordinary' and 'extraordinary' means of treatment. Our scrutiny will show that supporters of the sanctity-of-life view are not only advocating that doctors should sometimes intentionally terminate their patients' lives, but also that doctors should do so on the basis of the quality or kind of life in question.

As we saw in Chapter 1, those who speak of the sanctity of human life do not only hold that it is always absolutely wrong to take human life intentionally, they also hold—and this tenet is of course captured in the second prong of the SLP—that all human lives are equally valuable, and that it is impermissible to base life and death decisions on the quality of the patient's life.

There is considerable merit in demonstrating that supporters of the sanctity-of-life view are, in fact, making quality-of-life judgements. One reason is that this raises the charge of yet another inconsistency in their views; the other reason, and the more important one for the final part of this book, is to show that even the staunchest defenders of the sanctity-of-life view are implicit supporters of what I want to call a 'quality-of-life ethics'. I shall be arguing for such a quality-of-life ethics in Chapter 5, and whilst there may be disagreement as to the *content* of such a quality-of-life ethics, my general approach cannot be rejected out of hand—at least not by anyone who has been shown to make life and death decisions on the basis of the quality or kind of life in question.

How, then, do supporters of the sanctity-of-life view make quality-of-life judgements? They make them, I shall argue, in the guise of such distinctions as that between 'ordinary' and 'extraordinary' means of treatment. We encountered that distinction in Section 3.53, where I argued that the distinction between the withdrawal of so-called ordinary and extraordinary means does not mark a distinction between the intentional and the non-intentional termination of life. In the present chapter, I shall argue that the ordinary/extraordinary means distinction is typically employed to draw a distinction not between particular means of treatment, but rather between different lives: those lives that supporters of the sanctity-of-life view think are worthy of preservation, and those that they think are not.

This implicit shift to quality-of-life considerations has not escaped the attention of some observers of the scene[1] and it has been argued that the language of ordinary and extraordinary means should be abandoned and replaced by a more appropriate terminology. Robert M. Veatch, for example, suggests that we adopt the language of reasonableness and the patient's perspective, whereas Paul Ramsey opts for a 'medical indications policy' which, he holds, will better safeguard the equal value of all human life.[2]

But, as we shall see, even thinkers like Ramsey and Veatch do not believe that a patient's life must always be sustained. This raises the following question: Can the tenet that all human lives are equally valuable consistently be combined with the view that it is sometimes permissible to withhold a readily available life-sustaining means from some, and only some, patients? I think it cannot. From the equal value of human life follows 'vitalism', or the view that all lives must be prolonged equally regardless of whether such measures will benefit or harm a particular patient. Few supporters of the sanctity-of-life view are vitalists. But those who are not, those who move away from such objective criteria as a medical means' availability and efficacy in preventing death and adopt instead the language of benefits or burdens to a patient, adopt—explicitly or implicitly—a quality-of-life approach. There is no half-way house. Either we base life and death decisions on the broadly construed interests of the patient (in which case we opt for a quality-of-life ethic), or we are oblivious to the interests of the patient and consistently follow the principle that all human lives are equally valuable and inviolable: if some lives are prolonged by particular medical means, then it will be impermissible to refrain from prolonging others.

In Section 4.2, I shall examine some of the arguments to the effect that not all lives that can be prolonged need to be prolonged because the means necessary to keep a patient alive are 'extraordinary'. I shall show that such arguments are typically based on quality-of-life considerations. In Section 4.3, I shall look at some attempts to reformulate the distinction between ordinary and extraordinary

[1] Richard McCormick': 'To Save or Let Die: The Dilemma of Modern Medicine', *The Journal of the American Medical Association* 229 (1974), 172–6; Helga Kuhse: 'Extraordinary Means', 74–82; President's Commission for the Study of Ethical Problems in Medicine and Biomedical and Behavioural Research: *Deciding to Forego Life-sustaining Treatment* (Washington: US Government Printing Office, 1983), 82–91.
[2] Veatch: *Death, Dying and the Biological Revolution*; Ramsey: *Ethics at the Edges of Life*, 155.

means in terms that do not involve quality-of-life judgements. I shall show that the most plausible of these attempts rely, again, on quality-of-life considerations.

## 4.2  HOW ORDINARY MEANS BECOME EXTRAORDINARY

### 4.21  *The Equal Value of Human Life*

Before beginning the discussion of the distinction between ordinary and extraordinary means of treatment, let us briefly recall, from Chapter 1, the full scope of the Sanctity-of-Life Principle.

The SLP, as it underlies the practice of medicine, is absolute in its prohibition of the intentional termination of life, or euthanasia—be this by an action or an omission. As the Vatican's *Declaration on Euthanasia* puts it: 'By euthanasia is understood an action or an omission which of itself or by intention causes death, in order that all suffering may in this way be eliminated.'[3]

We have already seen, in Chapters 2 and 3, that a doctor's refraining from preventing death is always an instance of the intentional causation of death. This means that it is, according to the SLP, always absolutely prohibited deliberately and voluntarily to let a patient die. There is, however, another directly related sense in which the sanctity-of-life view is absolute as well: it makes no distinction between different kinds or qualities of human life—*all* human life is equally valuable.

The Vatican's *Declaration on Euthanasia* thus states that the absolute prohibition of the intentional termination of life encompasses the whole spectrum of human life from foetal life to the lives of those who are incurably ill or dying.[4] As we have already seen, Chief Rabbi I. Jakobovits confirms that this absolute respect for human life is shared by the Jewish tradition: human life, he says, is 'infinitely valuable', and it is morally irrelevant whether 'one shortens life by seventy years or only by a few hours, or whether the victim of murder was young and robust or aged and physically or mentally debilitated'.[5]

---

[3] Sacred Congregation: *Declaration on Euthanasia*, 6.
[4] Ibid., 7.
[5] As cited by Cardinal John Heenan, 'A Fascinating Story', 7.

Not all supporters of the SLP hold that life is infinitely valuable. Whilst the view that life is absolutely inviolable but not infinitely valuable has its own problems, this is not something I shall pursue. For our purposes it is sufficient to note that in the context of the sanctity-of-life doctrine, all human life is seen as at least equally valuable. The latter view is taken by the Protestant theologian, Paul Ramsey, whose views will be discussed in Section 4.3. As Ramsey puts it in a previously cited passage: 'All our days and years are of equal worth whatever the consequences; death is no more a tragedy at one time than at another time.'[6]

But if all our days and years are of equal worth, then it follows that a doctor must not refrain from preventing a patient's death, neither because the patient's life is of one kind or quality, rather than another, nor because death can be staved off for only a limited period of time. In the following, I include both length of life and quality or kind of life under the generic term 'quality or kind of life'; where distinctions are needed, I shall make these explicit.

With this, we have once again captured the Sanctity-of-Life Principle: '*It is absolutely prohibited either intentionally to kill a patient or intentionally to let a patient die, or to base decisions relating to the prolongation or shortening of human life on considerations of its quality or kind*'.

Here we are concerned with the second part of the SLP: that life and death decisions must not be based on qualitative considerations because all human life, regardless of its quality or kind, is equally valuable and has an equal claim to preservation. Bearing the prohibitory scope of the SLP in mind, we now turn to the distinction between ordinary and extraordinary means of treatment.

### 4.22 What Are Ordinary and Extraordinary Means?

The most natural understanding of the distinction between ordinary and extraordinary means of treatment is that of the difference between usual and unusual care, where 'ordinary' denotes what is statistically common or usual. This is an understanding based on current medical practices, and the one most commonly employed by physicians. Medically, 'extraordinary' thus tends to be identified with non-standard treatment, the new, and the rare.

Then there is the notion, also pervasive in the medical literature,

---

[6] Ramsey: *Ethics at the Edges of Life*, 191. See also Section 1.3.

that some care is 'simple' (or ordinary), whereas other care is 'complex' (or extraordinary), that is, elaborate or employing high technology and/or considerable effort.[7]

On either of these two interpretations, for example, the administration of antibiotics to fight off a life-threatening infection would now generally be regarded as ordinary treatment. On the other hand, a complex resuscitation method might be regarded as 'ordinary' according to the 'standard practice' understanding, whereas it might be regarded as 'extraordinary' according to most high technology interpretations.

As is fairly evident, on either of these two interpretations there will be borderline cases and disagreement as to whether a particular means is to be classified as 'ordinary' or 'extraordinary', since neither the usual/unusual nor the simple/complex interpretations of the distinction are marked by clear boundaries. This is, however, not the fundamental difficulty that marks these interpretations of the ordinary/extraordinary means distinction. The fundamental problem is not that of unclear borderline cases, but rather the failure of these understandings of the distinction to mark a difference in *moral relevance* between ordinary and extraordinary means. And yet, the distinction between ordinary and extraordinary means must be marked by such a morally relevant difference because ordinary treatment is deemed morally obligatory, whereas extraordinary treatment is not.[8]

It is quite obvious that the question as to whether treatment is common or unusual, or simple or complex, is in itself morally irrelevant when deciding whether or not such treatment ought to be employed. It is true that an unusual treatment may be less efficacious than a usual one; but if this is so, then it is *this* difference that is morally relevant in deciding for or against its employment. Similarly, a complex high technology procedure may be more costly than a simple one, and given the scarcity of medical resources, it would be *this* difference that is relevant to determining the allocation of resources. But it is also fairly obvious that there is no perfect correlation between these morally relevant features and the usual/unusual or the simple/complex distinctions; and to the extent that this

---

[7] See Albert R. Jonsen and George Lister: 'Life Support Systems', in Warren T. Reich (ed.): *Encyclopedia of Bioethics* (New York: Free Press, 1978), vol. ii, pp. 841–8.

[8] See, e.g., Pius XII, *Acta Apostolicae Sedis*, 49 (1957), 1031/2.

correlation is lacking, it is clear that the distinction between ordinary and extraordinary means is not, in these senses, morally relevant.[9]

But, as we have already seen in Section 3.53, in ethical analysis (as distinct from some of the medical literature), the distinction between ordinary and extraordinary means differentiates not between the usual/unusual or the simple/complex, but rather between what is 'ordinary' and 'extraordinary' in relation to a particular patient. In ethical analysis, the ordinary/extraordinary distinction separates what is regarded as morally obligatory treatment for a particular patient (ordinary treatment) from what is merely optional treatment (extraordinary treatment). To briefly recall our previous discussion, ordinary means are—according to the widely accepted definition of Gerald Kelly, SJ—all 'medicines, treatments and operations, which offer a reasonable hope of benefit for the patient and which can be obtained and used without excessive expense, pain or other inconvenience'. Extraordinary means, on the other hand, are 'all medicines, treatments and operations which cannot be obtained without excessive expense, pain or other inconvenience, or which, if used, would not offer a reasonable hope of benefit'.[10]

More recently, the Vatican's *Declaration on Euthanasia* has noted that whilst the distinction between ordinary and extraordinary means 'as a principle still holds good . . . some people prefer to speak of "proportionate" and "disproportionate" means'. Whatever the terminology used, the statement continues,

it will be possible to make a correct judgment as to the means by studying the type of treatment to be used, its degree of complexity or risk, its cost and the possibility of using it, and comparing these elements with the result that can be expected, taking into account the state of the sick person and his or her physical and moral resources'.[11]

All these factors—cost, availability, risk—are obviously highly morally significant. But just as no satisfactory correlation in morally relevant features marked the usual/unusual and the simple/complex interpretations of the ordinary/extraordinary means distinction, so no satisfactory correlation can be established between such objective factors as cost, availability, or risk of treatment, and traditional ascriptions of particular treatments as either morally obligatory or

---

[9] See also President's Commission: *Deciding to Forego Life-sustaining Treatment*, 82–90; and Kuhse and Singer: *Should the Baby Live?*, 30–7.
[10] Kelly: *Medico-moral Problems*, 129.
[11] Sacred Congregation: *Declaration on Euthanasia*, 10.

morally optional. Some treatments that pose no risk to life—treatments that are freely available and inexpensive and that would, if employed, predictably prolong the patient's life—are under certain circumstances considered 'extraordinary' or 'disproportionate', and hence non-obligatory. Even a simple injection of antibiotics may, under certain circumstances, be an extraordinary means. Such an injection is an extraordinary means, according to the traditional view, if it does not offer a 'reasonable hope of benefit'.[12]

### 4.23   Benefits, Burdens, and Quality of Life

This raises an obvious question: What constitutes a 'reasonable hope of benefit'? Quite clearly, medical treatments do not offer a reasonable hope of benefit if it is known that they will be efficacious neither in prolonging the patient's life nor in ameliorating her condition, or if the probability of their doing so is very low. But, again, this is not the way in which the distinction between ordinary and extraordinary means has traditionally been understood. What distinguishes ordinary from extraordinary means is not, for example, their efficacy in prolonging the patient's life, but rather their efficacy in prolonging a certain *quality or kind of life*.

We may see both Kelly's discussion of the distinction between ordinary and extraordinary means and the Vatican's subsequent discussion of the distinction in terms of proportionate and disproportionate means as embodying two sets of criteria for a medical treatment to be 'ordinary' or 'proportionate':

1. it must not involve excessive expense, pain or other inconvenience
2. it must offer a reasonable hope of benefit.

As Beauchamp and Childress correctly point out, the substance of the distinction is a balance between benefits and detriment, where it is assumed that the excessiveness or disproportionateness of treatment is determined by the probability and magnitude of the benefit.[13] Now generally speaking, life is a good, and to prolong life, or to prevent death, is to confer a benefit on a person. But putting the matter thus, it becomes apparent that the proportionateness or disproportionate-

---

[12] See, for example, Jonathan Gould and Lord Craigmyle (eds.): *Your Death Warrant? The Implications of Euthanasia* (London: Chapman, 1971), 91–3; The Linacre Centre Working Party: *Euthanasia and Clinical Practice*, esp. 57, 70; Haering: *Medical Ethics*, 146.

[13] Beauchamp and Childress: *Principles of Biomedical Ethics*, 118.

ness of a means will decisively be determined by what the patient's life will be *like* with or after treatment. Of course, if there is no reasonable hope that a given treatment will prolong a patient's life, then the effort may well be regarded as excessive. But this is not our central case. In the tradition we are discussing, even treatment that has a high probability of being efficacious in staving off death will, under certain circumstances, be described as extraordinary and non-obligatory. What we are left with, then, is an evaluation of the means in terms of the *magnitude* of the expected benefit—and it is here, I suggest, where quality-of-life considerations play a decisive role: the quality and quantity of the life in question will determine whether a particular means will be regarded as ordinary or extraordinary.

Take the case of a patient who, like Patient *F* in Section 3.52, is afflicted with terminal cancer, suffers great pain or discomfort, and contracts pneumonia. If the pneumonia were treated with antibiotics, such a patient could expect a few more weeks, perhaps months, of life. Without antibiotic treatment, it is expected that the patient will die within the next few days. If the doctor withholds antibiotic treatment, is she refraining from preventing death by ordinary or by extraordinary means?

Generally, supporters of the SLP hold that in a case such as this, antibiotic treatment is extraordinary and non-obligatory.[14] But why should this be so if we presuppose the belief that treatment would stave off pneumonia and that the patient could expect a further span of life? Doctors do not normally let their patients die of pneumonia by withholding antibiotic treatment. So why is it deemed permissible to withhold treatment in this case? What is abundantly clear is that in a case such as this, a simple course of injections is regarded as 'extraordinary' because the quality or kind of the patient's life, after treatment, is believed to be such that it ought not to be prolonged.

But if it is held that not every life that *can* be prolonged by readily available medical means need or ought to be prolonged, if the optionality or obligatoriness of treatment depends on whether it offers a 'reasonable hope of benefit' to the patient, then the distinction between ordinary and extraordinary means is based on quality-of-life considerations. A means can be either ordinary or extraordinary, depending on the medical condition of the patient and the kind of life available to her with, or after, treatment. Thus, it has been pointed out in the literature, the concept of 'extraordinary

[14] See n. 12

treatment' is extremely flexible. As James M. Gustafson puts it, 'under one set of circumstances a procedure may be judged ordinary, and under another extraordinary'.[15] Similarly, Bonnie Steinbock, as we have seen in Section 3.53, regards a respirator as 'ordinary' if it is used to sustain a patient through a severe bout of a respiratory ailment, but as 'extraordinary' if used to sustain the life of a permanently comatose patient.[16]

But in the case of the respirator as in the case of antibiotics, the term 'extraordinary' has been so relativized to the condition of the patient that it is precisely the condition of the patient that changes an ordinary means into an extraordinary one. The respirator and the antibiotics become extraordinary because the respective patients' quality of life is so 'extraordinary' that no life-sustaining treatment ought to be given.

A similar quality-of-life judgement is also implied in Bishop Lawrence Casey's support for the 1976 USA landmark decision to remove permanently comatose Karen Ann Quinlan from the respirator because

she has no reasonable hope of recovery from her comatose state by the use of any available medical procedures. The continuance of mechanical [cardiorespiratory] supportive measures to sustain continuation of her body functions and her life constitute extraordinary means of treatment. *Therefore, the decision of Joesph . . . Quinlan* [Karen's father] *to request the discontinuation of treatment is, according to the teachings of the Catholic Church, a morally correct decision.*[17]

Mechanical measures are extraordinary because, while they sustain Karen's life, they sustain it only in a comatose state. It is the comatose state which is determinant, not the inherent 'extraordinariness' of the means, nor the fact that Karen 'has no reasonable hope of recovery'. If the recovery criterion were decisive, then the continued use of iron lungs for polio victims and the continued injection of insulin for diabetics would also be extraordinary and hence optional because they do not lead to recovery from the state of paralysis, nor cure the diabetic condition. But all three forms of treatment have one

[15] James M. Gustafson: 'Mongolism, Parental Desires, and the Right to Life', in Robert F. Weir (ed.): *Ethical Issues in Death and Dying* (New York: Columbia University Press, 1977), 162.

[16] Steinbock: 'The Intentional Termination of Life', 72.

[17] 70 N.J. 10 In the Matter of Karen Quinlan, reprinted in Steinbock (ed.): *Killing and Letting Die*, 31 (emphasis in original).

thing in common: their continued application will prevent the patient's death. If it is thus permissible to refrain from preventing death in the one case but not in the other two, a defender of this view must point to a morally relevant difference that distinguishes these cases. It is not, as we have seen, an objective distinction between ordinary and extraordinary *means*, considered simply as means; and it is not the distinction between the intentional and the non-intentional causation of death. If there is a morally relevant difference between these two cases, it must lie elsewhere. And so it does: it lies not in the nature of the means, but in the different qualities or kinds of life preserved by those means.[18]

Quality-of-life considerations are also most obvious in discriminatory resuscitation practices. In 1982, the Medical Society for the State of New York issued its first guidelines for withholding emergency resuscitation from terminally ill patients whose heart or breathing fails. The guidelines describe the medical circumstances under which doctors may withhold potential life-prolonging medical treatment such as cardiopulmonary resuscitation: when in their judgement 'such so-called "heroic" emergency measures are not in the best interests of a dying patient'.[19] Thus death is not prevented in these cases if it is deemed that life will no longer be of any benefit to the patient.

Similar views govern the treatment of seriously handicapped infants. In a 1982 submission to the Law Reform Commission of Western Australia, the Australian Medical Association suggested that certain infants should be allowed to die if continued life is not in the infant's best interests:

It is the AMA's view that in certain circumstances, where doctors and parents agree that prolonging life would only prolong the baby's distress, it should be given no treatment other than to make it comfortable and allowed to die. Surely when it is deemed to be in the best interest of the child that its life should not be prolonged, the ability to refuse to prolong its life should exist.[20]

In its report *Deciding to Forego Life-sustaining Treatment*, the American President's Commission puts forward rather similar views

[18] See also the debate between myself and Gerald J. Hughes: 'Extraordinary Means', 79–82.
[19] News item: *New York Times*, 19 September 1982.
[20] Submission of the Australian Medical Association to the Law Reform Commission of Western Australia, June 1982, 18.

when it suggests that treatment may be foregone in situations where an infant's handicaps 'are so severe that continued existence would not be a net benefit to the infant'.[21]

Most remarkable, however, is the shift in the American Medical Association's position. In its 1973 policy statement, the AMA still relied on the distinction between ordinary and extraordinary means to justify the practice of letting some patients die. The AMA's 1986 policy statement no longer refers to means of treatment; instead it advocates an unambiguous quality-of-life approach:

> For humane reasons, . . . a physician may do what is medically necessary to alleviate severe pain, or cease or omit treatment to permit a terminally ill patient whose death is imminent to die . . . Even if death is not imminent but a patient's coma is beyond doubt irreversible . . . it is not unethical to discontinue all means of life prolonging medical treatment.[22]

Doctors, their medical associations, and ethics commissions are not alone in advocating quality-of-life standards. Rather, as my above discussion has shown, also supporters of the SLP base their arguments as to the obligatoriness or optionality of life-prolonging treatment on implicit quality-of-life considerations.[23]

Let me conclude the present section by citing just one more example of how quality-of-life considerations enter ethical reasoning expressed in terms of means of treatment. The theologian Leonard Weber extensively discusses the ethical issues raised by the birth of seriously handicapped infants in his book *Who Shall Live?*[24] Weber explicitly rejects the view that decision-making ought to be based on quality-of-life considerations. A quality-of-life ethic, he holds, offends against the equality of all human lives; the 'extraordinary-means approach', on the other hand, will offer some protection against an

> arbitrary decision being made on the basis of a judgment about the worth of a particular type of life. The decision will still be difficult and may still involve judgments about what constitutes successful treatment, but the focus on

---

[21] President's Commission: *Deciding to Forego Life-sustaining Treatment*, 218.

[22] The 1973 Statement is cited in full in Sect. 3.53. The 1986 Statement is dated 15 March 1986 and is available from the AMA's Council on Ethical and Judicial Affairs.

[23] On the optionality of resuscitating certain patients, i.e. instances when the means are 'extraordinary', see also Pope Pius XII, Address of 24 Feb. 1957, to doctors and surgeons in response to questions by anaesthetists, *Acta Apostolicae Sedis* 49 (1957), 1031–2.

[24] Leonard Weber: *Who Shall Live?* (New York: Paulist Press, 1976).

means is a constant reminder that we should not decide who should live or die on the basis of the worth of someone's life.[25]

What, then, is 'extraordinary treatment' according to Weber? For handicapped infants, Weber holds, treatment is extraordinary or non-obligatory when it does not offer a reasonable hope of success (i.e. that the child can be kept alive for more than a few days or weeks), if it imposes an excessive burden in terms of, for example, repeated surgical interventions; or if such treatment leaves the child seriously handicapped (for example, brain damaged). Here the following quotation will be instructive:

One can even talk about treatment imposing an excessive burden when it is the timing of the treatment that results in a burdensome life. If, for example, the oxygen supply to the brain has been stopped and the opportunity to resuscitate such a person only comes when it is probable that excessive damage has already been done to the brain, it should be considered an extraordinary means to attempt to restore normal blood circulation, no matter how common the procedure. By saving the life of the patient *at this time*, an excessive burden would be imposed . . . others would probably say that the decision not to treat in such a case is based on concern for the quality of the life of the child. And, of course, they are largely correct.[26]

However, despite his granting that others would largely be correct in saying that decisions such as these are based on quality-of-life considerations, Weber still wants to speak of such *treatment* imposing an extraordinary burden. As he puts it, the child 'would not have this burden if it were not for this treatment now'.[27]

Here I can do no better than state the objection raised by Richard A. McCormick to Weber's analysis. McCormick holds that the 'burden' Weber speaks of 'is precisely the damaged condition. It is *that* which is the basis for the decision. And if that is so, we are— regardless of the language we use—actually making quality-of-life judgments.'[28]

Faced with the decision to choose between life in a damaged condition (by, for example, resuscitating a brain-damaged infant) and death (by, for example, not resuscitating a brain-damaged infant), Weber implicitly suggests that there will be occasions when

[25] Ibid., 85.
[26] Ibid., 92–3 (my emphasis).
[27] Ibid., 93.
[28] Richard A. McCormick: 'The Quality of Life, the Sanctity of Life', *Hastings Center Report* 8 (1978), 34.

we should choose death for an infant. Why? Not because resuscitation procedures are an excessive burden (they are the same for normal and for brain-damaged infants), but because *life itself* would be such a burden for a brain-damaged infant—a burden that need not, or ought not, to be imposed on the infant.

I conclude, therefore, that as long as the distinction between ordinary and extraordinary means derives its moral significance from the proportionality of benefits and burdens for a particular patient, it will ineluctably be based on quality-of-life considerations: the same kind of treatment that is held to be beneficial for one person will be regarded as burdensome for another. Why? Not because there is a distinction in the treatment, nor because it will ward off death in one case but not in the other. Rather, treatment will be regarded as ordinary/extraordinary, proportionate/disproportionate, beneficial/burdensome, and so on, depending on the quality or kind of life in question: whilst a longer life will be of benefit to one patient, it will be a burden to another. However, to subscribe to *that* view is to subscribe to a quality-of-life ethics, and means the abandonment of the SLP: decision-making is based not on the equal value of all human life, but rather on the kind of life in question.

### 4.3 RECENT REFORMULATIONS OF THE ORDINARY/EXTRAORDINARY MEANS DISTINCTION

Some supporters of the sanctity-of-life view (as well as other people) have put forward proposals as to how the distinction between ordinary and extraordinary means might be redrawn. In the following, I shall discuss the most plausible of those views and shall attempt to show that here again the justification for a limited duty of life-preservation rests in quality-of-life considerations.

#### 4.31 *The Patient's Perspective*

Robert Veatch is one of the writers in the field who have recognized that the terms 'ordinary' and 'extraordinary' are extremely vague and are used inconsistently in the literature. He urges that they be banned from further use. Instead, he suggests, it will be clearer to simply speak of 'morally imperative' and 'morally expendable' means.[29]

To distinguish between morally imperative and expendable means, Veatch suggests that we adopt the patient's perspective, and what he

---

[29] Veatch: *Death, Dying, and the Biological Revolution*, 106 and 110.

calls the 'language of reasonableness'. Thus equipped, Veatch argues, we can determine what treatment it is reasonable to forego in the case of incompetent patients—namely, treatments the refusal of which 'would seem within the realm of reason to reasonable people'.[30]

Whilst such notions as 'usualness' and 'usefulness' are often relevant considerations in determining whether it is reasonable to refuse treatment, Veatch holds that even 'usual' treatments ought to be regarded as dispensable if they inflict a severe burden on a particular patient. Such thinking leads Veatch to the following conclusion:

A reasonable person would find a refusal unreasonable (and thus treatment morally required) if the treatment is useful in treating a patient's condition (though not necessarily life-saving) and at the same time does not give rise to any significant patient-centered objections, based on physical or mental burden; familial, social or economic concern; or religious belief.[31]

In the case of competent patients, other-directed concerns (such as burden to the family) are valid reasons for the patient to refuse life-prolonging treatment; in the case of incompetents, Veatch says, only patient-centred objections provide valid reasons for letting a patient die. Whilst it could be argued that the same standards should be applied to competent and incompetent patients as far as other-directed objections are concerned,[32] this is not a question I shall pursue. However, Veatch's analysis also raises a question of direct concern for our present purposes: Veatch speaks of morally required treatment for incompetents in terms of the treatment's usefulness in treating the patient's condition. What Veatch does not make clear, though, is how the term 'useful' is to be understood. We may consider treatment 'useful' if the treatment is not too burdensome and if it prolongs life. We may even consider extremely burdensome treatment 'useful' if, after treatment, we can expect to enjoy a good quality of life. And we may consider non-burdensome life-prolonging treatment as 'useless' if it leaves us with a life that is itself burdensome. Finally, is treatment 'useful' which will, as in the case of Karen Ann Quinlan, extend permanently comatose life?

The notion of 'usefulness' needs explication because it offers an implicit choice between a 'sanctity-of-life' and a 'quality-of-life' ethic. The point is that treatment may be 'useful' in prolonging life, but that

[30] Ibid., 110–12.
[31] Ibid.
[32] See, e.g. McCormick: 'The Quality of Life', 32–3.

a longer life is not always 'useful', or of benefit, to the patient: either because the patient is permanently comatose, or because life—with or after treatment—is excessively burdensome to the patient. If we therefore adopt the patient's perspective, as Veatch suggests we should, then treatment is 'useful' only if it either ameliorates the patient's condition or if it extends a life that is 'useful' or of benefit to the patient.

But to understand the notion of usefulness in this sense is also to adopt a quality-of-life approach: treatment may reasonably be foregone (and is therefore morally expendable) if it is useless in achieving a quality or kind of life that is of benefit to the patient. The alternative is the sanctity-of-life approach: to understand the notion of 'usefulness' in terms of a treatment's efficacy in prolonging life, irrespective of whether or not a longer life is of benefit to the patient. That approach, however, is in conflict with our adopting the patient's perspective: we can all imagine instances where life is so intolerable, so filled with suffering, so utterly without satisfactions, that we would not wish to live such a life and that it is reasonable to suppose that no one would.

In urging us to adopt the patient's perspective and the language of reasonableness, Veatch thus advocates a quality-of-life ethic: The life of an incompetent patient ought to be prolonged if it is in the patient's interest to have her life prolonged; it ought not to be prolonged if life is not in the patient's interest.

The position of Richard A. McCormick, a Catholic moral theologian, is similarly grounded.[33] Despite his religious affiliations, McCormick argues that the distinction between ordinary and extraordinary means relies on implicit quality-of-life considerations. However, McCormick also holds that the sanctity-of-life and the quality-of-life approaches ought not to be set against each other. Rather he suggests, 'quality-of-life assessments ought to be made within an overall reverence for life, as an extension of one's respect for the sanctity of life'. Whilst every person is, for McCormick, of 'equal value, not every life is'. Thus it is not unjust to provide discriminatory treatment: whilst it may be wrong to refrain from preventing one person's death, it may not be wrong to do so in another case. Inequality of treatment need not be unjust. Unjust discrimination is avoided, McCormick holds, if decision-making

---

[33] McCormick: 'To Save or Let Die', 172–6. *Idem*: 'The Quality of Life'.

centres on the benefit to the patient—even if that benefit is largely described in terms of quality-of-life criteria.[34]

McCormick is thus quite explicit in opting for a quality-of-life approach when the decision has to be made whether or not a particular patient's life ought to be prolonged by available means: it ought to be prolonged if continued life is of benefit to the patient; it ought not to be prolonged if the life open to the patient is a burden.

### 4.32   The 'Medical Indications' View

The Protestant theologian Paul Ramsey has noted with concern the implicit quality-of-life judgements also within the ranks of those purportedly subscribing to the sanctity-of-life view.[35] Opposing the view that any life and death judgements should be based on quality-of-life considerations, Ramsey urges that the 'cumbersome, opaque and unilluminating' terminology of the ordinary/extraordinary means distinction be abandoned. Instead, he suggests, we should adopt a 'medical indications policy'.[36]

When, then, is it permissible according to Ramsey to refrain from using an available life-sustaining means? That question, he says, can be answered by distinguishing between dying and non-dying patients. As far as the dying are concerned, Ramsey suggests, curative treatment is no longer indicated; the relevant choices are between further palliative treatment and no treatment. For non-dying incompetent patients, on the other hand, there is an obligation to use those means that are 'medically indicated'.[37]

In the absence of such a medical indications policy, Ramsey contends, we are moving toward active non-voluntary euthanasia for incompetent patients who are not dying. Against such developments, Ramsey asserts 'an undiminished obligation first of all to save life and, in the second instance, to use palliative treatment where this is possible'.[38]

Above all, Ramsey urges, quality-of-life judgements are to be avoided because they violate the *equality of human life*.[39]

---

[34] McCormick: 'The Quality of Life', 35. In his earlier article 'To Save or Let Die', McCormick advanced a different quality-of-life criterion: 'minimum personal relatedness'. If this criterion is not met, life need not be prolonged.

[35] Ramsey: *Ethics at the Edges of Life*, 145 ff.

[36] Ibid., 154–7, 172.

[37] Ibid., 160–81.

[38] Ibid., 165.

[39] Ibid., 191.

In the following, I will attempt to show that Ramsey's medical indications policy is untenable as a half-way house: not only is its terminology as unilluminating and opaque as that of the ordinary/ extraordinary means distinction which he rejects, but it also harbours implicit quality-of-life considerations.

*Karen Ann Quinlan*      In the light of Ramsey's medical indications policy, let us once again look at the case of Karen Ann Quinlan.[40] Permanently comatose Karen Ann Quinlan, it was believed, could be kept alive indefinitely with the help of a respirator, whereas she would die 'in a matter of minutes' if the respirator were switched off.[41] In a case such as this, Ramsey holds, it is permissible to refrain from preventing death because 'treatments that were potentially life-saving (or reasonably believed to be so) when first begun have now become means of aimlessly prolonging Karen's dying'. In other words, treatment may (according to Ramsey) be discontinued because it 'will affect the still living patient's condition in no significant respect except to prolong dying'.[42]

In arguing for the permissibility of refraining from preventing Karen Quinlan's death, Ramsey thus employs the distinction between dying and non-dying patients. Karen Quinlan is assigned to the category of the dying. This raises the fundamental question as to how we are to understand the distinction between dying and non-dying patients. Ramsey admits that he does not know when a patient is dying but that 'the reply must be that this is a *medical* judgment and that physicians can and do determine . . . the difference between dying and non-dying terminal patients'.[43]

But the judgement that someone whose life could be prolonged (indefinitely) by available medical means is 'dying' and therefore need not have her life prolonged is not a *medical* judgement; rather it is an *ethical* judgement as to whether, and if so when, it is permissible to refrain from preventing death. The case of Karen Ann Quinlan illustrates in a poignant fashion the conflation in Ramsey's analysis of value-free medical judgements and value-laden quality-of-life decisions. If 'dying' is to be understood in the value-free medical sense implied by Ramsey's analysis of the case—namely, that a patient is

[40] Paul Ramsey discusses this case in 'Prolonged Dying: Not Medically Indicated', *Hastings Center Report 6* (1976), 14–17; and in *Ethics at the Edges of Life*, 268–300.
[41] Paul Ramsey: *Ethics at the Edges of Life*, 268.
[42] Ramsey: 'Prolonged Dying: Not Medically Indicated', 16.
[43] Ramsey: *Ethics at the Edges of Life*, 187.

'dying' if she can survive only with the help of some medical means and is expected to die if this means is withdrawn—then those suffering from diabetes and from many other diseases would fall into this category of the dying, for whom only palliative or no treatment would be 'medically indicated'. And yet, nobody would seriously suggest that a diabetic patient is, other things being equal, dying, and that no further life-prolonging treatment ought therefore to be administered. What is clear is this: if 'dying' is understood as the medical judgement that death will occur *if and when* treatment is withheld or withdrawn, then the concept is useless for ethical analysis because it does not tell us when treatment may justifiably be withdrawn and when it ought to be continued.

The position is similar with regard to the second possible interpretation of the dying/non-dying distinction we can glean from Ramsey's statement: that it is permissible to withhold treatment from those patients whose condition will not significantly be affected by the treatment, that is, that treatment may be withheld if it does not cure or ameliorate the patient's underlying medical condition. As Ramsey puts it, 'if it will affect . . . the patient's condition in no significant respect except to prolong dying'.

It might be thought that treatment is effective only if it leads to recovery (the state of health or well-being enjoyed by the patient prior to her medical condition), or at least to a partial recovery. But if *this* is the notion Ramsey has in mind—and it is difficult to know whether he has, since he does not give content to many of his crucial terms—then the term 'recovery' would already imply a certain quality of kind of life, over and above a medical treatment's efficacy in staving off death, and would, other things being equal, infringe the equality of all human life. Moreover, we have already seen in Section 4.2 that it is not necessary for a treatment to cure or improve a patient's underlying condition for it to be routinely administered; an iron lung to sustain a polio-victim and insulin for a diabetic patient illustrated the point. So, again, the distinction between treatment significantly affecting/not affecting the patient's underlying *medical* condition will not allow us to distinguish between those patients who are dying and those who are not.

Since Ramsey does not provide any other criteria as to how we might distinguish between dying and non-dying patients, this leaves him with two options. Either all those patients who require medical assistance to sustain life and/or those whose medical condition cannot be improved by medical means beyond keeping them alive are 'dying' and need not have their lives prolonged; or alternatively, if Ramsey wants to hold that the patients in this group are not dying, then neither is Karen Ann Quinlan, and it will be impermissible to refrain from preventing her death. To distinguish the case of Karen Ann Quinlan from other similar cases, Ramsey relies on implicit quality-of-life considerations. This becomes apparent when he says that Karen's treatment may be discontinued because 'no treatment is *beneficial* to a comatose . . . patient'.[44] But the judgement that a treatment is beneficial over and above prolonging her life is not an objective *medical* judgement, rather it is a value-laden quality-of-life judgement. So what Ramsey is saying is that it is permissible to refrain from preventing Karen's death not because she is dying or incurable, but because treatment is no longer of any benefit to her. However, whilst it is indisputably true that a permanently comatose patient can no longer benefit from any treatment, the judgement that treatment may therefore be withdrawn and the patient let die is also indisputably a quality-of-life judgement: treatment may be withdrawn because, whilst it sustains life, it sustains only a certain quality or kind of life, a kind of life that is no longer of any benefit to the patient.

*Handicapped infants*  Implicit quality-of-life considerations also form the backbone of Ramsey's 'medical indications policy' for handicapped newborn infants.[45] Once again, Ramsey's analysis depends on distinguishing between those patients who are dying and those who are not. However, whereas in the case of Karen Ann Quinlan the 'dying' were those who required medical support and would die without it (and/or those whose medical condition would not 'significantly be affected' by treatment), in the case of defective infants Ramsey employs a different notion of the dying. The dying, Ramsey holds, are those infants who 'cannot be helped', that is, those infants who will die *irrespective* of the medical treatment administered. Non-dying infants, on the other hand, are those who are expected to live if they are treated 'as medically indicated'.[46]

This appears to be a plausible way of distinguishing between those patients who are dying and those who are not, and one that would

[44] Ibid., 269 (my emphasis).
[45] Ibid., 181–267.
[46] Ibid., 181–8.

initially seem to avoid medical vitalism on the one hand and quality-of-life considerations on the other. As we shall see, though, this initial plausibility is deceptive.

From the distinction between those infants who are dying and those who are not, Ramsey derives different treatment policies. As already noted, curative treatment is, according to Ramsey, no longer indicated in the case of the dying and ought to be replaced by a policy of palliative treatment or no treatment. In the case of non-dying infants, on the other hand, 'medically indicated' treatment ought to be administered. What treatment, then, is 'medically indicated' for those infants who are not dying? Ramsey does not expressly state the conditions that make a treatment medically indicated; instead he refers us to the treatment policy advocated for spina bifida infants by R. B. Zachary, a paediatric surgeon at the Children's Hospital in Sheffield, England.[47] In the practices of R. B. Zachary, Ramsey sees 'decisive proof that the relentless use of all medical means is *not* the only alternative to a routine use of the distinction between ordinary and extraordinary means or to admitting the entrance of a quality-of-expected life policy into medical practice'.[48]

As we saw in Section 2.2, when children are born with spina bifida, one or more of the spinal vertebrae have failed to close completely. The spinal cord and nerves in that area, which normally control muscles and sensations in the bladder, bowels, and legs, may bulge through the opening in the bone and form a fluid filled sac protruding from the child's back. Because the sac is often only partly covered by a fragile membrane, the unprotected nerves are easily damaged and the risk of paralysis and infection is high. However, by operative means the spinal cord and nerves can often be tucked back into the vertebral column and the skin closed over the opening; this improves the infant's survival chances markedly.[49]

As Paul Ramsey recounts the practice of R. B. Zachary, there are two groups of spina bifida infants on whom Dr Zachary does not perform the operation to close the lesion on the infant's back. One

[47] Ibid., 181–7. The contrasting policy of Zachary's colleague, John Lorber, was briefly discussed in Ch. 2, Sect. 2.2. Zachary's views are put forward in various articles, e.g., R. B. Zachary: 'The Neonatal Surgeon', *British Medical Journal* 4 (1976), 866–9; and 'Ethical and Social Aspects of Spina Bifida', *Lancet* 2 (1968), 274–6.

[48] Ramsey: *Ethics at the Edges of Life*, 182.

[49] In addition to the literature already cited, see also C. A. Swinyard: *Decision Making and the Defective Newborn: Proceedings of a Conference on Spina Bifida and Ethics* (Springfield: Charles C. Thomas, 1978).

group consists of infants whose wound is not suitable for the operation, that is, the wound is such that it *cannot* be closed by surgical means. The second group of infants on whom Zachary does not operate consists of those infants who are expected to die 'within a few days or weeks'. Treatment is withheld, Ramsey writes, because the infants are 'dying', not because the operation should be classed as either 'ordinary' or 'extraordinary', or because there is a prognosis of long-term dysfunction. 'None of the babies in this group', Ramsey holds, 'should be operated on because to do so would have no bearing on whether it lived or died. No one can help them; there is no obligation to try and do the useless.'[50]

However, whilst an operation is clearly useless in the first group of babies on whom Zachary does not operate, in what sense is it 'useless' in the second group—in the case of those babies who are expected to die within a few days or a few weeks? Will these babies die within a few days or weeks because the operation is useless in the sense of being inefficacious, or useless in only prolonging the infants' lives by a certain period of time over and above the short span of life expected for them? It is clearly the second sense of 'useless' Ramsey has in mind, because he holds that in the case of those patients that are identified as dying no further attempts should be made to *prolong* their lives by available medical means.[51]

This raises questions about both the process of dying and about the uselessness or futility of life-prolonging treatment for those patients identified as dying. Let us take these notions in turn.

Ramsey's analysis critically depends on drawing a distinction between dying and non-dying patients, because only this distinction will allow him to avoid vitalism on the one hand and quality-of-life considerations on the other. But when is a patient such as a newly born infant dying? This, Ramsey says—as we have already noted—is a medical judgement. And so it is. It is a medical judgement that a patient suffers from a certain terminal illness and can be expected to die from it within a few days, weeks, months, or years. But it is *not* a medical judgement to hold that because a person is afflicted with such a terminal condition and is expected to die at *some* future date, her death ought not *now* to be prevented if it can. Let me elaborate.

As a first move, however, we must sharpen our focus. Ramsey does not say how Zachary identifies those spina bifida infants 'born

[50] Ramsey: *Ethics at the Edges of Life*, 182–3.
[51] Ibid., 187, 192.

dying'—whether they are thought to be dying because they are afflicted with a particular form of spina bifida, or because they are also afflicted with some other terminal condition that is expected to lead to their early deaths. That the cases can be substantially different will be intuitively obvious. In the first case the infant's life could possibly be prolonged by an operation and other vigorous treatment, whereas in the second case the question as to whether or not such an infant's life could be prolonged by an operation or some other treatment would depend on how soon death from the terminal condition could be expected, whether the likelihood of her dying from the terminal illness first is greater than the probability of her dying from an infection if left unoperated, and so on. Undoubtedly, in the real world of the intensive care nursery, matters are even more complex. What is certain, though, is that much *factual* uncertainty surrounds ethical discussions relating to the treatment of spina bifida infants. Such factual uncertainty begins with the various criteria employed by different physicians to select infants for treatment or non-treatment, it surrounds the efficacy of varying treatments in different hospital settings, and it extends to the long-term and short-term survival rates of infants selected according to different criteria and subjected to different treatments or non-treatments by different doctors.[52] Because ethical analysis presupposes clarity about the facts of the matter to which it addresses itself (and because a detailed examination of the medical literature to establish such medical facts would divert us too far from our present goal), I shall examine the distinction between dying and non-dying patients in another medical context in which it will be easier to agree on the facts of the situation.

In addressing himself to the distinction between dying and non-dying patients, Ramsey discusses another case which meets the requirement of greater factual clarity: Tay-Sachs disease, a hereditary disorder that mainly affects infants of Jewish ancestry. In Tay-Sachs disease an infant appears normal at birth but is, as Ramsey puts it, 'born destined to die'.[53] Some time after birth, infants afflicted with this disease develop an extreme sensitivity to noise, muscle weakness, and a cherry-red spot appears on the highly sensitive area near the centre of the retina. Progressive loss of vision eventually results in blindness. There is severe mental deficiency. Affected children

[52] See n. 49.
[53] Ramsey: *Ethics at the Edges of Life*, 191.

generally die at about three years of age. There is no cure for Tay-Sachs disease.

However, whilst such Tay-Sachs children are 'destined to die', Ramsey holds that 'pre-symptomatically [they] are not dying any more than the rest of us are'. Let me quote Ramsey at some length, thereby also stating once more his views on the equal value of all human life:

For the first six months approximately [a Tay-Sachs baby] is like any other baby; living and growing and presumably enjoying human existence as any other infant would. In religious perspective there is no reason for saying those six months are a life span of lesser worth to God than living seventy years before the onset of irreversible degeneration. A genuine humanism would say the same thing in other language. It is only a reductive naturalism or social utilitarianism that would regard those months of infant life as worthless because they lead to nothing along a time line of earthly achievement. All our days and years are of equal worth whatever the consequence; death is no more a tragedy at one time than at another time. When the symptoms of irreversible degeneration show themselves and the child is in the throes of its very own dying, investigational therapies—including the search for a cure at high risk to an afflicted child—are quite in order. But from some point in the dying of Tay-Sachs children they ought not to be stuck away in Jewish chronic disease hospitals and have their dying prolonged through tubes. The ethics of only caring for the dying holds without any modulation or modification in the case of a child no less than in that of an adult terminal patient who has entered upon the process of dying. No treatment is indicated when none exists that can do not more than prolong dying.[54]

On the one hand, Ramsey seems to be saying that life is somewhat more valuable (to God) before the onset of irreversible degeneration (because at this time life should presumably be sustained) than it is after the onset of such degeneration (when life should no longer be sustained). On the other hand, Ramsey appears to be saying that *all* our days and years are of equal worth 'whatever the consequence', that is that all life—degenerate or not—is equally valuable and has an equal claim to preservation.[55] It is clear, though, that Ramsey must, in theory, subscribe to the second position: were he to advocate the first, he would be subscribing to a quality-of-life ethic. And yet, the *practical* recommendations Ramsey makes as far as the treatment of

[54] Ibid., 191–2.
[55] On the equal value of human life and its equal claim to preservation, see ibid., 168–9.

the 'dying' and 'non-dying' patients is concerned appear to be based on the first position. Let me show why.

These apparently irreconcilable views of life being/not being equally valuable are given the semblance of some initial plausibility by Ramsey's equivocation on the words 'useless' or 'futile' treatment, and his distinction between 'dying' and 'non-dying' patients. A Tay-Sachs baby, after the age of approximately six months, enters the 'dying process'. Now, it is obvious that treatment ought not to be administered to the dying (or to anyone else) if it is believed that the treatment is inefficacious in either ameliorating the patient's distress or in prolonging life. But not all treatments that can be administered to the 'dying' are 'useless' or 'futile' in this sense. Rather, there are many treatments that will prolong the patient's life, even if they do not, in any way, affect the patient's underlying terminal condition. Once again, antibiotic treatment is an obvious example. Let us assume that a Tay-Sachs baby, after it has entered the 'dying process' at approximately six months, contracts bronchitis at age nine months. Since it is a severe bout of bronchitis, it is believed that the infant will die if antibiotic treatment is withheld. According to Ramsey's analysis, is it permissible—or even obligatory—to withhold antibiotic treatment? The answer is not clear, for Ramsey merely suggests that 'from some point' in the dying process these infants should not have their lives prolonged. What is clear, though, is that *if* it were decided that antibiotic treatment should not be administered and if, as a consequence, the infant dies, then the infant did not die from untreatable Tay-Sachs disease, but rather from treatable but untreated bronchitis. In other words, the child would have been *allowed to die*.

Now, Ramsey does not say at what point in the dying process it is permissible to withhold life-prolonging treatments such as anti-biotics. But he holds that there *is* such a point. The reasoning underlying Ramsey's analysis appears to be this: whilst a Tay-Sachs baby enjoys life like any other infant during the first six months of its life, there is a considerably decreased level of enjoyment (or no enjoyment) some time after the onset of irreversible degeneration. When this point has been reached, we should no longer sustain the infant's life, because life is no longer of any benefit to the infant. In other words, the infant should be allowed to die on the basis of quality-of-life considerations.

On the surface of his analysis, Ramsey avoids quality-of-life considerations by distinguishing between 'dying' and 'non-dying' patients. However, it is not only that it will be difficult to devise a generally acceptable (physiological?) definition of dying, it is fundamentally Ramsey's failure to provide any arguments as to why the distinction should have moral significance that renders his position untenable. It may well be that a person with, say, Parkinson's disease starts the process of irreversible degeneration at age thirty-five, and has a further life-expectancy of twenty years, which is marked by a continual decline. However, even if such an irreversible process of degeneration can be identified medically, and even if we were to agree to say that such a person were 'dying', this does not mean that it would therefore be morally permissible for a doctor to refrain from preventing death. As far as Tay-Sachs infants are concerned, Ramsey holds that 'from some point in the dying process' they ought not to have their lives sustained. However, whilst suggesting that such a point exists somewhere along the continuum of the dying process, Ramsey does not say when this point will be reached, how it is to be identified, or why that point should be morally relevant. What is clear, though, is that *wherever* this point lies, its location cannot be determined by a 'medical indications policy'—for the point Ramsey has in mind is not the point when an infant would be dying irrespective of what is done, but rather that point at which we should stop *prolonging the infant's life*.

In connection with the 'non-dying', Ramsey holds that certain treatments are medically indicated: those that are efficacious in achieving a desired result such as closing a lesion; those that are routinely administered to normal infants; and those that will enhance bodily human life and prevent its deterioration.[56] It will be clear that treatments that meet these conditions will also be 'medically indicated' for the 'dying' if quality-of-life decisions are to be avoided. The point is that the 'dying' are not in the 'throes of their very own dying', as Ramsey puts it, if the decision is made to withhold treatment that would, if applied, prolong their lives. They will be in the throes of their own dying only if there is nothing the doctor can do to prolong life, that is, when she does not refrain from preventing death. Whenever a doctor refrains from preventing death, the patient dies not from an incurable and ultimately fatal disease, such as Tay-Sachs disease, but from some secondary curable disease, such as bronchitis. When such an infection could be combatted with

[56] Ibid., 182–3, 187, 192.

available antibiotics, if such antibiotics are routinely applied in the case of 'non-dying' infants, and if such treatment would be expected to enhance (prolong?) the patient's bodily life and prevent its deterioration, then such treatment would be medically indicated. If the decision is made that such treatment ought not to be employed because the patient is 'dying', then such a decision will ineluctably be based on quality-of-life considerations.

Take an example from the recent report of a Catholic Working Party on *Euthanasia and Clinical Practice*. The members of this working party are intent, like Ramsey, on avoiding quality-of-life judgements in medical decision-making. Like Ramsey, they are also aware of the fact that the ordinary/extraordinary means distinction poses a difficulty for supporters of the SLP in just this respect.[57] Inspite of these difficulties, the report suggests that it is not necessary 'to be troubled by ambiguities attaching to the terms "ordinary" and "extraordinary". It is the underlying considerations determining when treatment is obligatory which are important.'[58]

I find it difficult to disagree because these underlying considerations are, as we shall see, precisely those quality-of-life considerations that the working party is trying so hard to avoid, and whose explicit discussion is indispensable if medical decision-making is to be based on an ethically sound footing.

Like Ramsey, the members of the working party 'decide'— although more explicitly—when a patient is dying and when she is not. This becomes apparent in the following example of the working party, designed to illustrate the circumstances under which a doctor may let a patient die. This example is, incidentally, discussed under the heading 'Patients with a lethal condition for which there are no life-saving treatments'.

A man in his late 50s had been in hospital for 8 years on account of advanced Parkinson's disease. During the last years of his life he lost weight progressively, became generally weaker and spent more time in bed. He was less able to talk clearly and needed increasing help with the basic 'activities of daily living'. During this time he had three attacks of bronchitis. The first two were treated with chest physiotherapy and antibiotics. In anticipation of a further attack, *it was decided* that the man was in fact dying, albeit slowly, and that the next episode of bronchitis would not be treated with physiotherapy and antibiotics but simply symptomatically on the grounds that curative treatment of the chest infection would, at this stage, be little

---

[57] Linacre Centre Working Party: *Euthanasia and Clinical Practice*, 46–8, 58.
[58] Ibid., 46.

more than 'resurrecting the man to die again a few weeks later', or 'prescribing a lingering death'. The outcome of a chest infection in these circumstances was quite likely to be the man's death and it was seen as the natural terminal event of the progressive physical deterioration.[59]

In the light of my above discussion, I believe this example speaks for itself and requires no further comment—except perhaps this one: that the working party had amongst its members at least one professor of Philosophy, Elizabeth Anscombe, and one Reader in Law with a special interest in natural law ethics, John Finnis.

Whether or not Ramsey would agree with the 'decision' of the working party that the patient in the above example was 'dying', I have no way of knowing. What is clear, though, is that his position— irrespective of his judgement on this particular case—is untenable: either he must subscribe to vitalism—the view that all human life that can be prolonged must be prolonged equally, irrespective of its quality or kind—or he must accept that judgements that it is sometimes permissible to refrain from preventing death will ineluctably be based on quality-of-life considerations. This is born out by Ramsey's own medical indications policy: if all treatments that are 'medically indicated' ought to be employed, irrespective of the quality or kind of life in question, we have vitalism. If 'medically indicated' treatments are sometimes not to be employed, we have a quality-of-life ethic: medically indicated treatments need not be employed if life-prolonging treatment, or continued life, is of no benefit to the patient. And the latter is not a medical judgement, but a value judgement based on the quality or kind of life in question.

While other arguments might be considered as to how the distinction between ordinary and extraordinary means might be reformulated, it is perhaps unnecessary to do so because it seems sufficiently clear that whatever form these attempts take, they will offer a choice between the SLP (or vitalism), on the one hand, and a quality-of-life ethics on the other. To the extent that even supporters of the sanctity-of-life view are not totally oblivious to the consequences that treatment decisions will have for the patient, they will adopt a quality-of-life approach. But that approach, of course, cannot consistently be combined with the SLP which regards all human life as equally valuable. In the context of the SLP, quality-of-life questions cannot even be raised: as Ramsey puts it approvingly when outlining R. B. Zachary's medical indications policy for spina

[59] Ibid., 56–7 (my emphasis).

bifida infants: 'Whether life will be beneficial to its possessor is not a question Dr Zachary asks.'[60]

However, even if this is a question supporters of the SLP do not openly ask, it is a question they ought to ask. Whilst such distinctions as those between ordinary and extraordinary means lend an initial plausibility to the claim that deciding not to prolong life in all cases is compatible with the SLP, reliance on such means-related distinctions also constitutes an abrogation of moral responsibility: that kind of moral responsibility that is associated with our sometimes having to choose death on the basis of explicit (and therefore morally defensible or indefensible) quality-of-life considerations. By presenting value-laden quality-of-life decisions as value-free medical decisions, substantive moral issues are evaded. Here the important point (to be substantiated in the concluding chapter) is this: we are faced not merely with a theoretical confusion, of interest only to philosophers and moral theologians, but with a misleading doctrine that has indefensible practical consequences as well.

[60] Paul Ramsey: *Ethics at the Edges of Life*, 187.

# 5

# Conclusion: From 'Sanctity-of-Life' to 'Quality-of-Life'

The preservation of life must be the sole principle guiding medical practice, including the treatment of the hopeless cancer patient. This principle cannot be tampered with or interpreted loosely.

> C. S. Cameron: *The Truth About Cancer*, 1956

It does sound quite barbarous for the doctor to kill his patient. It seems improper. But it is also improper to force a suffering patient, who has long been deteriorating, who is dying or already dead, to continue to vegetate. That must be made uncommon. It is always barbarous.

> J. H. van den Berg, MD: *Medical Power and Medical Ethics*, 1978

Sir, In his well-written and beguiling paper, Mr Zachary makes out a good case for treating all babies with severe spina bifida surgically, yet Dr Sanders describes this as 'shallow and cruel', to which Mr Zachary retorts that the alternative is to kill these babies. . . . There is, of course, a third approach—namely to let Nature take its course. Over the years, without any active intervention on my part, over 90% of the untreated babies I have seen have died before their first birthday.

> Ian G. Wicks: *The Lancet*, 1968. Ian Wicks is here referring to R. B. Zachary's article: 'Ethical and Social Aspects of Treatment of Spina Bifida', *The Lancet*, 1968, and to subsequent letters to the Editor of the same journal

If a patient is worth working on, the only way to work on him is flat out. If there is even a small chance, give him full support—but don't give just enough support to let him die slowly. . . . A patient is worth treating outright—or not at all. Half treatment is a terrible way to let a patient die.

> Dr Christopher Bryan-Brown, as cited by Jane J. Stein: *Making Medical Choices*, 1978

A man who killed the woman he loved because she was dying from cancer was sent to a mental hospital for an indefinite period. . . . The judge told Searby: '. . . She was enduring terrible physical misery but she had a right to live. Her misery could well have been discounted by your love. I will not accept that you killed her out of affection. Love doesn't kill life, it supports it.'

*Daily Telegraph*, 1972

To fight a human being to death, to try him, condemn him to death and execute him, are grave and tragic actions. But they may be compatible with this awe and respect [for human life]. To kill him (whether he is oneself or someone else) because one judges his life wretched or not worth living, is not.

Working Party: *Euthanasia and Clinical Practice*, Linacre Centre 1982

## 5.1 INTRODUCTION

SUPPORTERS of the Sanctity-of-Life Principle find repugnant and depraved the view that it may sometimes be morally right to terminate life intentionally on the basis of quality-of-life considerations. And yet, as my discussion in previous chapters has shown, not only is refraining from preventing death always an instance of the intentional termination of life, but the qualified Sanctity-of-Life Principle is also based on quality-of-life criteria whenever the withdrawal or non-employment of life-prolonging means is justified by the implicit or explicit claim that those means would not benefit the patient over and above prolonging her life. If ethical analysis is not totally oblivious to the benefits and burdens accruing to the patient, then it is difficult to see how quality-of-life judgements can be avoided.

Of course, implicit quality-of-life judgements in the arguments of those purportedly subscribing to the sanctity-of-life view are not always based on benefits and burdens to the *patient*. Rather, they might also be justified by appealing to burdens accruing to the family (or society), not only from the treatment but also from the quality or kind of life that would be open to the patient after treatment. As Pius XII put it in his address of 24 February 1957 to doctors:

The rights and duties of the [patient's] family depend in general on the presumed will of the unconscious patient if he is of age and *sui generis*. As to the family's own independent duty, the only obligation in normal circumstances is to employ ordinary means. Consequently, if it were to appear that the attempt at resuscitation constitutes in truth a burden on the family such as one could not in conscience impose on them, they can legitimately insist that the doctor cease his attempts, and the doctor can legitimately comply. In this case there is *no direct disposal of the life of the patient, no euthanasia, which would never be permissible;* even when it brings about the cessation of circulation, the interruption of the attempts at resuscitation is only ever indirectly a cause of the cessation of life.[1]

In previous chapters, I have argued that the qualified SLP is internally inconsistent because it is based on morally and conceptually untenable distinctions; in the present chapter, I shall argue that the qualified SLP ought to be rejected because it is not only a theoretically confused principle, but one that has unacceptable consequences in practice as well. Here I shall primarily focus on those arguments that are implicitly based on benefits and harms to the patient. It is obvious, however, that the difficulties for supporters of the SLP would be compounded if account were also taken of their frequent failure to distinguish adequately between the interests of the patient and the interests of her family, or society at large, when life and death decisions are made on the basis of the quality or kind of life in question. Clearly, the difference between a stance according to which the features that make an action right depend on the welfare of the patient herself and one in which they depend on the consequences for others as well is a crucial one, and one that needs to be made explicit. This is, however, a problem that I shall not pursue. For our purposes it is sufficient to restrict the discussion to the framework of benefits and burdens to the patient because the SLP excludes quality-of-life considerations as bases for decision-making, irrespective of their grounding.

Nowadays, few supporters of the Sanctity-of-Life Principle are 'vitalists', that is, supportive of the view that a patient's life must be prolonged even if continued life is not of benefit to the patient, or in her best interests.[2] However, to the extent that supporters of the SLP are not 'vitalists', but rather hold that a patient's life need not be prolonged if life with or after treatment is expected to be excessively burdensome, then they are advocating the intentional termination of life, and are doing so on the basis of the quality or kind of life in question.

---

[1] *Acta Apostolicae Sedis* 49 (1957), 1032.

[2] As Joseph Fletcher puts it bluntly ('Euthanasia', in Joseph Fletcher: *Humanhood: Essays in Biomedical Ethics* (Buffalo, NY: Prometheus Books, 1979), 150): 'Ethically, the issue whether we may let such a patient go is as dead as Queen Anne . . . The last serious advocate of this unconditional provitalist doctrine was David Karnofsky, the great tumor research scientist . . . The issue of *negative* euthanasia is settled ethically.' (I have quoted David Karnofsky in Ch. 1, n. 22.)

If my arguments in the preceding chapters have been correct, the qualified SLP is fatally flawed because it both prohibits and condones the intentional termination of life. What is more, those who hold that it is sometimes permissible to cause a patient's death intentionally are typically supporting their life and death judgements by implicit quality-of-life criteria. This means that there are convincing theoretical reasons for rejecting the SLP as an internally inconsistent principle—a principle which does not meet the formal requirements of consistency outlined in Section 1.6. In addition, there are also strong practical reasons for rejecting the SLP: in being theoretically confused, the qualified SLP leads to muddled practice and to ethically indefensible consequences.

In the preceding chapters, I have provided the theoretical grounds for rejecting the qualified SLP. I take these arguments as given. Section 5.2 will therefore be descriptive: it will illustrate the practical muddles and inconsistencies that seem unavoidable if those involved in ethical theorizing and medical decision-making continue to subscribe to the view that it is always impermissible intentionally to cause death, and that quality-of-life judgements can be avoided by focusing on means of treatment. In approaching the question of the justifiable termination of life in terms of means of treatment, rather than in terms of the quality or kind of life in question, substantive moral issues are evaded: issues that relate to the locus of the value of human life, and to the question as to why it is sometimes, but not always, wrong intentionally to shorten it.

In Section 5.3, I shall provide a brief sketch as to how arguments might proceed to the conclusion that it is sometimes permissible to take life intentionally on the basis of the quality or kind of life in question. I present this tentative outline both to eliminate the temptation to deal with the vexing ethical issues of terminating life in the oblique and often inappropriate manner of the ordinary/ extraordinary means criterion (or any other means-related criterion); and to show that if doctors may in some cases justifiably refrain from preventing death on the basis of quality-of-life considerations, then positive euthanasia is often morally preferable to letting patients die.

## 5.2  INDEFENSIBLE PRACTICAL CONSEQUENCES

When a patient is allowed to die earlier than she otherwise would because death is thought to be preferable, from her point of view, to life with or after treatment, we are dealing with a case of negative euthanasia: death is regarded as the morally preferable option, and the patient is allowed to die for her own sake.

For the moment, let us assume that such judgements are unproblematic in that whenever it is thought to be permissible to refrain from preventing death, an earlier death is indeed the desirable outcome for the patient. However, even if we accept this assumption, what is highly problematic is the judgement that it is morally preferable to withhold or withdraw treatment from such patients who are deemed to be better off dead, rather than to kill them quickly and painlessly by, say, administering a lethal injection.

To illustrate the point, let us once again look at the example of a man dying from Parkinson's disease. This case, it will be remembered, is presented by a prestigious Catholic working party on euthanasia as an example of a permissible instance of letting die.[3]

The working party assumes—albeit implicitly—that it is in the patient's best interest to die because he is facing a 'lingering death'. In the light of this judgement, the decision is made that the next bout of bronchitis is not to be treated with antibiotics and physiotherapy and that the patient should be allowed to die.

But the practice of choosing death in this implicit way is undesirable for two main reasons: firstly, it may involve patients in much unnecessary suffering; and, secondly, it may lead to decision-making being made on morally irrelevant grounds. Let me deal with these two points in turn.

John Lorber, who pioneered the selective non-treatment of spina bifida infants, notes the undesirable consequences of negative euthanasia. In Lorber's study, sixty per cent of untreated infants died before they were one month old, and none lived for more than eight months.[4] But isn't even one month, a week, or a day, too long if it involves much suffering for these infants? Lorber seems to agree when he writes: 'It is painful to see such infants gradually fading away over a number of weeks or months when everybody hopes for a speedy end.'[5]

To shorten the dying process of an infant selected for non-treatment, Lorber advocates (as we saw in Section 2.2) that 'nothing

---

[3] Linacre Centre Working Party: *Euthanasia and Clinical Practice*, 57; for the description of the case, see Sect. 4.32.
[4] Lorber: 'Ethical Problems', 55.
[5] Ibid., 58.

should be done which might prolong the infant's survival'. In particular, doctors should resist the temptation to operate because 'progressive hydrocephalus is an important cause of early death'. Lorber thus sees clearly that it is better for an untreated infant to die early rather than fade away over a number of weeks or months. He also recognizes that to distinguish between positive and negative euthanasia in these cases might well involve 'a major inconsistency and perhaps hypocrisy'.[6] Despite this recognition, however, Lorber also holds that even if positive euthanasia were legal, he would 'certainly never do it'.[7] In this, I take him to be appealing to something like the qualified SLP: that a doctor may sometimes let die, but must never take positive steps to bring about an infant's death.

To see what may happen when the decision has been made to let an infant die, let us look at the case of a Down's syndrome infant born with an intestinal obstruction. As we have previously seen, when discussing Case *E* in Section 3.52, in such circumstances it is frequently decided to refrain from performing a routine operation to remove the obstruction, with the foreseen consequence that the infant will die. One paediatric surgeon, Anthony Shaw, describes the dying process in the following way:

> When surgery is denied, the doctor must try to keep the infant from suffering while natural forces sap the baby's life away. As a surgeon whose natural inclination is to use the scalpel to fight off death, standing by and watching a salvageable baby die is the most emotionally exhausting experience I know. It is easy at a conference, in a theoretical discussion, to decide that such infants should be allowed to die. It is altogether different to stand by in the nursery and watch as dehydration and infection wither a tiny being over hours and days. This is a terrible ordeal for me and the hospital staff—much more so than for the parents who never set foot in the nursery.[8]

Whilst there may have been changes in the way in which infants are allowed to die since Anthony Shaw wrote the above passage in 1972, it is nonetheless true that negative euthanasia can be a terrible ordeal for all involved—not least the infant for whose sake, we assume, doctors and parents are engaging in the practice of euthanasia in the first place. The tragedy is, of course, that patients, relatives, and medical staff undergo these ordeals on the basis of a distinction that

[6] Ibid., 54, 55, 57.
[7] Lorber: 'Commentary I and Reply', 121.
[8] Antony Shaw: 'Doctor Do We Have a Choice?' *New York Times Magazine*, 1972, p. 54, as cited by Rachels: 'Euthanasia, Killing and Letting Die', 159.

is, in itself morally irrelevant: the distinction between killing and letting die, or positive and negative euthanasia.

Both positive and negative euthanasia are instances of the intentional causation of death, and whilst it is true that killing is often worse than letting die, what makes it worse in those cases are factors extraneous to the distinction. However, even if it is agreed that killing is, in actual fact, often worse than letting die, this admission will not be helpful to a supporter of the qualified SLP for the problem at hand. As we have seen, in arguing for the permissibility of letting die, supporters of the qualified SLP implicitly base their judgements on the quality-of-life premiss that the patient would be 'better off dead'. But if the patient would be 'better off dead', then to kill her would often serve her interests better than to let her die.[9] This also means that the agent who kills the patient for the patient's sake is, other things being equal, not a worse kind of agent than the agent who lets the patient die for the patient's sake, and may be a better kind of agent in all those cases where killing serves the interests of the patient better than letting die. With this, the residual basis of the PDE disappears: even if an agent who aims at the death of a person because she wants her dead is often a bad kind of agent, this is not the case in all those cases where death is in that person's best interests.[10]

Take the case of the patient suffering from Parkinson's disease. In this case, there are three options:

1. The first option is 'vitalism', the view that the patient's life has the same value as that of other patients and must be prolonged by efficacious means, even if a longer life will not benefit the patient. In this case, the patient's bronchitis and other complications will be treated, and the patient will have a few more weeks or months of a 'lingering death' before he finally dies of Parkinson's disease or one of its untreatable complications.

2. The second option, advocated by the Catholic Working Party on Euthanasia, and the one generally taken to be implied by the

---

[9] Space will not permit me to discuss here the philosophical difficulties involved in comparing existence with non-existence, or in ever rationally choosing non-existence. I take it, however, that there will clearly be situations where death is not only the preferred option, but also the one which it is rational to choose for oneself or another. (See, for example, Bernard Williams: 'The Makropulos Case: Reflections on the Tedium of Immortality', in James Rachels (ed.): *Moral Problems*, 2nd. edn. (New York: Harper & Row, 1975), 410–28, esp. 414; in the same volume, Thomas Nagel: 'Death' 401–9.

[10] See Ch. 2, n. 99.

qualified SLP, is to refrain from treating the patient with antibiotics and physiotherapy if and when the next bout of bronchitis occurs. In this case, the patient will linger on until the opportunity presents itself to let him die of a treatable but untreated infection.

3. The third option, and the one strongly opposed by all supporters of the SLP, is to administer a painless lethal injection when the stage has been reached where life is no longer of benefit to the patient. In this case, the patient will die at once and there will be no lingering dying process.

Those who oppose the intentional termination of life in all its forms argue that we must take the first option. As one doctor, C. S. Cameron, put it some thirty years ago: 'The preservation of life must be the sole principle guiding medical practice, including the treatment of the hopeless cancer patient.' For Cameron, there is no difference between positive and negative euthanasia. He regards the distinction between euthanasia and letting the patient die by omitting life-sustaining treatment as a 'moral quibble'.[11] In this, I suggest, Cameron is right.

The view that life must be prolonged even if life presents an intolerable burden to the patient is so patently cruel that simply to state the position will amount to its rejection as a plausible ethical principle. Medicine would become not only a zealous but also a callous discipline—where, in the spirit of the sanctity of all human life, every flicker of life would have to be prolonged by 'furore therapeutics', surgery, and resuscitation: doctors would, in the language of the Catholic Working Party on Euthanasia, be 'prescribing a lingering death' and 'resurrecting' the dying. Whilst such a position seems so patently inhumane that few of us would want to defend it, it is consistent with the Sanctity-of-Life Principle's two tenets: that all human life is equally valuable and absolutely inviolable. The principle's inhumanity and its disregard for the interests of individual patients is the price one has to pay if one wants to subscribe to the view that it is always wrong intentionally to terminate life on the basis of quality-of-life considerations. I suggest the price is too high.

In the light of the patent inhumanity of 'vitalism', it is the qualified SLP, positing a limited duty of life-preservation in certain cases, that

[11] C. S. Cameron: *The Truth about Cancer* (Englewood Cliffs, NJ: Prentice Hall, 1956), 115–16.

needs to be attacked, because it is *this* principle which is widely supported and whose practical implications are unacceptable. Let us look at this principle, exemplified by option 2 above, in the context of the patient suffering from Parkinson's disease.

The rationale for letting the patient die earlier than he otherwise would is that he is facing a lingering death: negative euthanasia is thought to be justified because continued life is judged not to be in the patient's best interests. The implicit reason for letting the patient die is thus that he would be 'better off dead'. But after having made this judgement, and after allowing that in circumstances such as these death ought not to be opposed, those purportedly having the welfare of the patient in mind opt for an often slow and distressing method of bringing death about: they let the patient die. The second position, consistent with the qualified SLP, is thus an untenable halfway house: whilst it holds—implicitly—that decision-making ought to be based not on the sanctity of human life but on the patient's interests, it decrees that whilst the patient need not linger on for weeks or months, he must nevertheless linger on in a state judged worse than death for a few more days or weeks until sooner or later and quite independently of human design or agency, he is afflicted with a potentially lethal (if untreated) disease that allows those supporting the qualified SLP to let him die. This is not only inconsistent with the reasoning that led to the decision to let the patient die in the first place (i.e. that the patient would be better off dead), it is also an abrogation of moral responsibility: whilst the patient has been marked for death, whether, and if so when, he will die is left to 'nature acting'. This approach must be rejected as constituting what Jean Paul Sartre would have called an act of 'bad faith', and as one that may involve particular patients in much unnecessary distress and suffering. If it is in a patient's interest to die because continued life is excessively burdensome, then positive, not negative euthanasia is—other things being equal—the morally preferable option.

Take another case, that of a Down's syndrome infant born with an intestinal obstruction. In a case like this, the infant cannot take fluid and food orally. If an operation is not performed, the infant will die by an often slow process of withering away, involving starvation, infection and, if intravenous fluids are withheld, dehydration. In the much-discussed Johns Hopkins case, the dying process took fifteen days.[12] The suffering involved in this is difficult to justify; indeed, it

[12] See, e.g., McCormick: 'The Quality of Life', 35.

seems clear that given the decision that death was, in this case, the morally preferable option, positive euthanasia, that is, option 3 above, would have better served the interests of the infant.

Here it may, of course, be objected that we cannot approach the question of the Johns Hopkins case in this light; it may be argued that doctors and parents were wrong to let the infant die. Given routine care, the argument might go, most mongoloid infants will lead happy, even if somewhat truncated, lives; the claim that it is in such an infant's interest to die can thus not be sustained. I have two comments on this.

So far, we have assumed that *whenever* the decision is made to let a patient die, death would be in the patient's best interest. But even if death were *not* in the patient's best interest, it would still be the case, other things being equal, that positive euthanasia would, in the cases we have discussed, be the morally preferable option (because more economical of suffering, and so on), once the decision has been made to refrain from preventing the patient's death.[13]

The underlying question is, of course, *whether* death is in a patient's best interest—but that question obviously cannot be tackled head-on by supporters of the SLP. The SLP prohibits the intentional termination of life, and affirms the equal value of human life. This means that life and death decisions can hence be made only obliquely—for example, in the guise of a 'means'-related language. However, what is oblique and merely implicit needs to be made explicit if decision-making is not to be based on morally irrelevant and indefensible grounds. How decision-making will come to be based on morally irrelevant grounds was already seen in the case of the patient suffering from Parkinson's disease. In the practice of letting some (and only some) Down's syndrome infants die slow and distressing deaths, the inadequacies of the qualified SLP become quite apparent.[14]

What we have in the qualified SLP is a principle that says that it is never permissible intentionally to kill a patient, but that it is

[13] See H. Kuhse: 'Death by Non-feeding: Not in the Baby's Best Interests', *Journal of Medical Humanities and Bioethics* 7:3 (1986).

[14] In the case of spina bifida infants, selective non-treatment may have another bad consequence: some infants will survive without treatment, but will now be worse off than they would have been had they received the appropriate treatment soon after birth. If the intention of non-treatment was that the infants should not survive because an early death was in their interests, their survival is a failure of the non-treatment policy. See John Freeman: 'The Short-sighted Treatment of Myelomeningocele: A Long-term Case Report', *Pediatrics* 53:3 (March 1974), 311–13.

sometimes permissible to refrain from preventing her death as long as the latter decision is a means-related one and not based on the quality or kind of life in question. But this is where the confusion comes in, because judgements that it is sometimes permissible to withdraw or withhold life-prolonging means are, in fact, based on quality-of-life criteria that are unarticulated and obtuse. When the decision is made to let certain Down's syndrome infants die by not performing a simple operation to remove an intestinal obstruction, this decision is procedurally indistinguishable from the decision to let the patient suffering from Parkinson's disease die of bronchitis. In both cases, life-sustaining treatment is withheld because death is thought to be the preferable outcome on account of the patient's underlying medical condition: Parkinson's disease and Down's syndrome, respectively. In the case of Down's syndrome infants, this means that those infants who happen to be born with an intestinal obstruction will be let die, whereas those who do not happen to have such an obstruction will live on. This means that here, as in the case of the patient suffering from Parkinson's disease, life and death decisions are based on morally irrelevant natural contingencies. But to leave things up to Nature rather than to rational human choice is, as Joseph Fletcher never tires of arguing, not truly human.[15]

The point that medical decision-making is frequently based on irrelevant grounds is also made by James Rachels, who puts the matter thus:

If you think that the life of such a [Down's syndrome] infant is worth preserving, then what does it matter if it needs a simple operation? Or, if you think it better that such a baby not live on, then what difference does it make if its intestinal tract is *not* blocked? In either case, the matter of life and death is decided on irrelevant grounds. It is the mongolism, and not the intestine, that is the issue. The matter should be decided, if at all, on *that* basis, and not be allowed to depend on the essentially irrelevant question of whether the intestinal tract is blocked.[16]

What is at the base of practices such as these is the qualified SLP which holds that when there is a potentially lethal condition, the patient may sometimes be allowed to die by withholding certain medical means; if there is no such condition, the patient will live on, for killing is always absolutely wrong. What has, however, not been examined by this means-related approach is whether or not the lives

[15] See, e.g., Joseph Fletcher: 'Recombining DNA', in Fletcher: *Humanhood*, 194.
[16] Rachels: 'Euthanasia, Killing and Letting Die', 160.

of Down's syndrome infants or of patients suffering from Parkinson's disease ought or ought not to be preserved. That question needs answering first. Only when it has been answered in the negative, will the question of method arise: whether the patient's life ought to be ended negatively or positively.

The important point is this: in continuing to subscribe to the qualified SLP, supporters of this view are not only adhering to an inconsistent principle, but to one that has indefensible consequences in practice as well. Much of the current medical literature shows that there has been an implicit shift to quality-of-life standards,[17] and sociological studies indicate how certain qualitative factors enter into medical decision-making in life and death cases.[18] But from the ethical perspective, the quality-of-life question is not adequately treated until and unless one gives morally relevant reasons as to why a certain quality or qualities *should* be decisive in terminating or continuing life-prolonging treatment. The sanctity-of-life doctrine, in denying the moral relevance of quality-of-life considerations, cannot raise these questions on a theoretical level. In practice, this means that the medical profession is, in the absence of such standards, faced with an anarchy of values and meaning. On the one hand, doctors have thus allowed a mongoloid infant requiring routine surgery to die by dehydration and starvation over a fifteen-day period on the grounds that surgery constitutes an extraordinary means,[19] and they have resuscitated six times, against his expressed wishes, a sixty-eight-year-old doctor suffering from terminal cancer on the grounds that resuscitation is now a standard procedure in the modern hospital setting.[20] They will do so without being able to say what value or values they are trying to serve other than to act in accordance with the qualified SLP—which holds that it is always impermissible intentionally to terminate life on the basis of quality-of-life considerations, but which also holds that it is sometimes permissible to refrain from preventing death.

By presenting quality-of-life decisions as an almost technical question (namely, as one concerning 'means' which may or may not be optional), substantive moral issues are evaded. One of these is the

[17] See the literature cited in Sect. 2.2.

[18] Diana Crane: *The Sanctity of Social Life: Physicians' Treatment of Critically Ill Patients* (New York: Russell Sage Foundation, 1975).

[19] McCormick: 'The Quality of Life', 35.

[20] See Case Study 14 in Beauchamp and Childress: *Principles of Biomedical Ethics*, 263–4.

question of what it is that we value when we decide—as in the case of permanently comatose Karen Ann Quinlan—that 'heroic intervention is not worthwhile'.[21] To decide that medical intervention is 'not worthwhile' requires a clear assessment of the locus of the value of human life, and if it derives from different sources, of their relative weights. As long as such substantive criteria are not made explicit, as long as we rely on the extremely flexible language of 'means' to make a sanctity-of-life ethic superficially credible, we will engage in muddled practice—and we will do so in the name of an ethic which affirms the equal value of human life but which does not, indeed cannot, ask whether the interests of a patient are better served by a longer or a shorter life.

What has made quality-of-life questions so pressing is that in our age of sophisticated medical technology, death is often not a natural, inevitable event. It is often only when supportive measures are withheld or withdrawn that death becomes inevitable. Discontinuing or not instigating such measures is unavoidably the intentional causation of death. It also requires, unavoidably, the shouldering of moral responsibility—not only for allowing death to occur sooner than it otherwise would, but also for doing so on the basis of the quality or kind of life in question.

Let me here provide a sketch (and it is only a sketch, since a full explication and defence of the view I am putting forward would require a book rather than a single chapter)[22] as to how reasoning based on quality-of-life considerations might proceed. I shall provide this sketch for a quality-of-life ethics in the context of the medical condition we have repeatedly encountered throughout this book: spina bifida.

## 5.3 SKETCH OF A QUALITY-OF-LIFE APPROACH

According to the secular version of the sanctity-of-life doctrine, it is always wrong intentionally to terminate human life because all human life is equally valuable and absolutely inviolable. As we saw in Chapter 1, here '$X$ is an innocent living human being' entails in conjunction with the SLP: 'It is absolutely wrong intentionally to

[21] B. D. Colen: *Karen Ann Quinlan: Living and Dying in the Age of Eternal Life* (Los Angeles: Nash, 1976), 115, as cited by Steinbock: 'The Intentional Termination of Life', 72–3.

[22] For my views on the treatment of handicapped infants, see: Kuhse and Singer: *Should the Baby Live?*

terminate $X$'s life.' In other words, human life is taken to be an intrinsic good, irrespective of whether it is of value to its possessor. I have two brief comments on this.

Firstly, we have already seen that merely to assert that the termination of human life is wrong because the state of being alive is itself intrinsically valuable barely rises to the level of an argument for the inviolability of human life, for it simply asserts that there is value in what the taking of life takes away. While it is true that it may be difficult to refute someone who consistently holds that mere human life, irrespective of its quality or kind, is intrinsically valuable, such a view is not apparent in the practice of medicine, nor in the arguments of those who allegedly subscribe to the sanctity-of-life doctrine. Moreover, and this brings me to my second point, it is a view both implausible and unattractive to all those of us who regard certain kinds of life as in no way preferable to death. Take the case of permanently comatose Karen Ann Quinlan: from the subjective point of view, there appears to be nothing to choose between permanently comatose existence and death. Arthur Schopenhauer made the point in the following way:

for the *subject*, death itself consists merely in the moment when consciousness vanishes, since the activity of the brain ceases. The extension of the stoppage of all other parts of the organism which follows this is really already an event after death. Therefore, in a subjective respect, death concerns only consciousness.[23]

And just as death, for the subject, consists merely in the moment when consciousness vanishes, so life consists, for the subject, in the presence of those conscious states that cease with the moment of death. Thus, a more plausible view than the one underlying the sanctity-of-life doctrine would appear to be this: whilst it is true that before there can be any subjective human experience or consciousness, there must be life, life is nonetheless only a condition for other human values and experiences. 'Human life' can thus mean different things: it can mean the existence of vital processes and metabolic functioning without any conscious states ('mere life'), and it can mean the life of an experiencing subject in the sense of a conscious or self-conscious human being.

These senses do not always overlap. If we understand the term

[23] A. Schopenhauer: *The World as Will and Representation*, trans. E. J. F. Payne (New York, 1969); as cited by Glover: *Causing Death and Saving Lives*, 45.

'human being' or 'human life' in the first sense, then the comatose patient, like the foetus conceived of human parents, is 'human'. If we understand it in the sense of an experiencing subject, the permanently comatose patient is no longer a human being, and the early foetus may be only a potential one. Joseph Fletcher has compiled a list of what he calls 'indicators of humanhood', which includes such characteristics as self-awareness, self-control, a sense of the future, a sense of the past, and so on;[24] and Robert Veatch suggests that the capacity to experience and the capacity for interaction are essentially significant to the nature of man.[25] I do not want to discuss these suggestions in detail, other than to note that the term 'human life' spans different notions: life that is biologically human ('mere life'), and conscious or self-conscious human existence. Do we want to say that all these 'lives' have equal value? And what would such a view entail?

### 5.31   What's Special About Human Life?

We have already noted that even those who speak of the 'sanctity of life' do not take their rhetoric seriously. In various ways, quality-of-life considerations enter into their life and death decisions. We should, however, also remind ourselves of our earlier discussion of the sanctity-of-life doctrine in Section 1.3. There we noted that those who speak of the 'sanctity of life' do not really mean to say that *all* life is sacred or has the same value. It is *human* life which they see as sacred; they are not generally saying that the life of a sheep, chicken, earthworm, or lettuce has the same value as the life of a human being. While this may seem quite obvious, we should keep this fact in mind because it will remind us that even those who want to rank all *human* life equally are making different judgements about the value of different lives.

But what *is* it that gives value to human life, but not—or not to the same degree—to the lives of other living things? Two answers are possible. The first answer is that human life has sanctity simply because it is *human* life, that is, because it is the life of a member of the species *Homo sapiens*. The second answer is that human life has special value because humans are self-aware, rational, autonomous,

---

[24] J. Fletcher: 'Indicators of Humanhood: A Tentative Profile of Man', *Hastings Center Report* 2 (1972), 1–4.
[25] Robert M. Veatch: 'The Whole-brain-oriented Concept of Death: An Outmoded Philosophical Formulation', *Journal of Thanatology* 3 (1975), 13–30.

purposeful, moral beings, with hopes, ambitions, life-purposes, ideals, and so on—roughly, that human beings are 'human' in Joseph Fletcher's sense of the term. Any of these qualities, or a combination of them, could serve as a basis for a moral distinction between human beings and lettuces or chickens. That such distinguishing qualities are needed is clear: for if the value of life were based on 'mere life', rather than on one or more of the above characteristics, then every life— including the earthworm's or the lettuce's—would be equally valuable.

It is not difficult to see that the second answer does point to a morally relevant difference between some lives and others. For example, it is quite plausible to hold that the life of a self-aware, rational, purposeful being that sees itself as existing over time is more valuable than the life of an entity or being who lacks these characteristics. But if one takes this approach, then one is not saying that human *life* has sanctity, but rather that rationality, the capacity to be self-aware, moral or purposeful, and so on, have 'sanctity'. Of course, one may still hold, as we noted in Section 1.3, that human life has sanctity or special worth, but only in so far as it is a precondition for rationality, purposiveness, or whatever else one takes the valuable characteristic to be. One would *not*, on this view, be able to argue that the lives of all members of the human species have special value—for example, the lives of the irreversibly comatose, or the lives of severely brain-damaged new-born infants. The second approach, then, does not give us a reason for preserving all human lives, and cannot serve as the basis for the view that *all* human lives, irrespective of their quality or kind, are equally valuable.

The first answer covers all human beings—by definition. But can the fact that a being belongs to the species *Homo sapiens* rather than to any other species tell us anything about the value of that being's life? I believe the answer is 'no'. The value of human life, and the wrongness of taking it, must not rest on 'speciesism'—namely, the view that human life has special value, simply because it is human life.[26] While it may initially seem obvious that human life is more valuable than non-human life, it is also 'obvious' to the racist or sexist that a persons's race or sex should determine how that person ought to be treated. But just as race or sex are not morally relevant in themselves, neither is species. If we say that the lives of beings of our own species are valuable, but the lives of beings of other species are

[26] See Singer: *Practical Ethics*, esp. Ch. 4.

not, *merely because these beings do not belong to our species*, then on what basis can we criticize the racist who says that the lives of members of her race have special value, but the lives of members of other races do not?

We may also approach that matter from yet another perspective. Imagine that we found that there are intelligent beings living on Mars. Whilst these beings do not *look* like us, they are self-aware, rational, autonomous, purposeful, moral beings, who care about their lives, the lives of others, and about their world. Would we not want to say that the wanton killing of such beings is wrong and reject as spurious the defence of a shooting party from Earth that they have done nothing wrong because these beings are, after all, not members of our species? I believe that neither race nor species are morally relevant in themselves. What matters are a being's capacities—the kind of life a being has.

This conclusion should, in my view, also be applied to decision-making in the practice of medicine. What is important is not that a patient is human (and therefore should have her life sustained). Rather, we must ask questions about the *quality* and *kind* of the patient's life.

## 5.32 Quality of Life and Interests

I start with the assumption that conscious life has value because it enables the existence of pleasurable states of consciousness.[27] Whilst the existence of pleasurable states is not the only value to which human life gives rise, it will be agreed, I think, that it is at least *a* value that morality ought to take into account. In other words, I am suggesting that life is not an intrinsic good, not a good in itself, but rather a means to something else—for example, pleasurable states of consciousness.

If we were thus to agree that the value of life is not in life *qua* life ('mere life'), but rather has its locus in the value it has for the individual concerned, then it would follow that life is not an unconditional good, but good only in so far as it is of value to its possessor. This means that not all life is equally valuable, as the sanctity-of-life view suggests, nor is it, as I want to suggest, always inviolable. To the extent that we can all envisage situations where we would choose death for ourselves rather than continue living, there will also be situations where any morality based on the Golden Rule

[27] See H. Kuhse: 'Interests', *Journal of Medical Ethics* 11 (September 1985), 146–9.

or the principle of-universalizability would direct that a moral agent take the life of another rather than preserve it.[28] What I am suggesting, then, is that there is a strong connection between the value of life and the interests of the being whose life it is. Life may be in a being's interests, or it may not—depending on what the life is like.

The view that life can be of value or disvalue to its possessor is apparently also taken by a number of influential bodies. The World Medical Assembly,[29] the United States President's Commission,[30] and the American Medical Association[31] have recently suggested that life and death decisions in the practice of medicine should be based on the 'best interests' of the patient. As the American Medical Association puts it in its 1986 Policy Statement, entitled *Withholding or Withdrawing Life Prolonging Medical Treatment*: 'In the absence of the patient's choice or an authorized proxy, the physician must act in the best interests of the patient.'[32] In other words, doctors are no longer vaguely exhorted to 'respect human life' as the 1948 *Declaration of Geneva* told them to;[33] rather, they are asked to act, other things being equal, in their patients' best interests, either by sustaining life or by refraining from doing so.

But when is life, or death, in a patient's best interests? To answer that question, it is important to distinguish not only between different *qualities* of life (lives, for example, that are filled with irrelievable suffering and lives that allow for pleasure or happiness), but also between different *kinds* of life—such as the lives of normal adults and the lives of newly born infants and foetuses.

Let me begin by describing a frequent practice: the practice of terminating a pregnancy if it is found that the foetus is abnormal and suffers from a defect, such as spina bifida.

When we offer pregnant women a test to see whether they are carrying a child with spina bifida, with the intent of making abortions available to these women if the test is positive, we are—explicitly or

---

[28] See, e.g., R. M. Hare: 'Euthanasia: A Christian View', *Philosophic Exchange* (1975), 43–52; also Hare: *Moral Thinking*, esp. 177 ff.

[29] World Medical Assembly: 'Statement on Terminal Illness and Boxing' 35th Medical Assembly, Venice, Italy, October 1983, *Medical Journal of Australia* 140 (October 1983), 431.

[30] President's Commission: *Deciding to Forego Life-sustaining Treatment*.

[31] American Medical Association: *Withholding or Withdrawing Life Prolonging Medical Treatment*, Statement of the Council on Ethical and Judicial Affairs, 15 March 1986.

[32] Ibid.

[33] World Medical Association: *Declaration of Geneva*.

implicitly—subscribing to a quality-of-life ethics. We are distinguish-ing between the life of the woman and that of the foetus. We are saying that foetal life and adult human life are of a different kind; and we draw from this the practical conclusion that different kinds of human life may be treated differently. We would all agree, I think, that the life of the pregnant woman—even if she were to suffer from spina bifida—is such that it must not, against her wishes, be terminated by doctors. Our practices suggest that foetal life may—at least sometimes—be terminated in the practice of medicine. On this view, then, we are saying that not all lives that are biologically human are the same: we are putting a wedge into the concept of human life, and are, in our practices, distinguishing between different kinds of life: foetal life and the lives of those who are 'human' in, for example, Fletcher's sense of the term.

A quality-of-life ethic, as it is implicit in prenatal testing pro-cedures and the subsequent availability of abortions, thus dis-tinguishes between different kinds of life and regards kind of life as relevant to the wrongness of taking life.

The question is, though, whether a quality-of-life ethics as implicit in these practices is defensible. I believe it is, although I shall here but hint at its content.

During the last few years, a number of philosophers have attempted to distinguish between different kinds of life and to establish principles relevant to action: what makes the taking of some but not all lives wrong?[34]

Michael Tooley has provided detailed arguments as to the foundation of what he calls a 'right to life'.[35] For him, the ability to see oneself as existing over time (also, of course, one of Joseph Fletcher's 'indicators of humanhood') is a necessary condition for the possession of a right to life, or the direct wrongness of killing.

I believe Tooley's argument is basically sound. The underlying principle of his argument is that the wrongness of an action is related to the extent to which the action prevents some interests, desires or preferences from being fulfilled. This basic principle explains both why it is wrong, other things being equal, to inflict pain, and why it is wrong, other things being equal, to kill a being with a desire to go on

---

[34] See, e.g., Glover: *Causing Death and Saving Lives*; Singer: *Practical Ethics*; John Harris: *The Value of Life* (London: Routledge and Kegan Paul, 1985); Rachels: *End of Life*.
[35] Michael Tooley: *Abortion and Infanticide* (Oxford: Clarendon Press, 1983).

living. Any being capable of feeling pain can have a desire that the pain cease; but only a being capable of understanding that it has a prospect of future existence can have a desire to go on living, and only a continuing self can have an interest in continued life. Tooley suggests that we reserve the term 'person' for those beings who are capable of understanding that they are continuing selves; and for the remainder of this section I shall be using the term 'person' in this way.

According to Tooley's analysis, neither human foetuses nor human infants, nor humans with severe mental retardation or brain damage, are persons; and it would not be directly wrong (that is, a wrong done to them) to take their lives. On the other hand, chimpanzees might be persons, and so might be some other non-human animals as well. Thus the notion of a 'person' as employed by Tooley, reflects no arbitrary species-based boundary, but characteristics of obvious relevance to the taking of life and the infliction of pain and suffering.

A quality-of-life ethic would, in my view, have to take account of principles such as the above. It would entail that the direct wrongness of killing lies not in taking life, but rather in overriding in a most profound way the interests, desires, and preferences of a person who does not want to die. This will have profound implications for decision-making in the practice of medicine.

### 5.33   Choosing Death

As we have seen throughout this book, the question is not *whether* decisions to end human lives should sometimes be made; rather, the question is on what principle or principles these inevitable life and death decisions should be based. This view was also taken by the Royal Dutch Association of Medicine when, in recommending that medical practitioners should be allowed to practise both positive and negative voluntary euthanasia, they held that the question was not whether or not euthanasia should be allowed—since it was already being practised—but rather when and how it should be practised.[36]

I have already suggested that we need to distinguish between those patients who are 'persons' in Tooley's sense of the term and those who are not, because these two groups of patients have different kinds of lives and interests. We now need to take the question of interests a step further and ask what it entails for medical decision-making.

[36] KNMG (Royal Dutch Association of Medicine) 'Policy Statement on Euthanasia', *Medisch Contact* 39:31 (3 August 1985).

*Competent patients and autonomy*     All patients capable of experiencing states of consciousness have an interest in well-being—that is, in freedom from pain or suffering, restoration of functioning, and so on. But in addition to that, normal adult patients ('persons') also have an interest in their own future—in controlling and shaping their lives, and in acting as autonomous moral agents. In other words, I am suggesting that there are two main values to which human life gives rise: pleasurable states of consciousness—the value I posited earlier on in this section—and the value of autonomy or self-determination, the latter linked in a fairly obvious sense to both Tooley's concept of a 'person' and to some of Fletcher's 'indicators of humanhood'.

At the very basis of medical decision-making there is thus a tension. It has its source in the difference between respecting the freedom or liberty of patients and securing their well-being. How is this tension to be resolved? We should begin, I believe, with the principle espoused more than a century ago by John Stuart Mill in his classic essay *On Liberty*.[37] Mill urged that the only legitimate basis on which the state may coerce the individual is to protect others: the individual's own good, whether physical or mental, is not sufficient warrant.

Whilst we might not want to regard this principle as an inflexible rule in all areas of life, I believe it ought to be the determinate one in the practice of medicine where life and death decisions for seriously ill or incapacitated patients are at issue. This conclusion has apparently also been reached by the Royal Dutch Medical Association when they suggest that the crucial question in euthanasia decisions is whether the patient wants to die on the basis of what *she* regards as unbearable suffering.[38] I share the Association's view, and believe that competent and informed patients should be allowed to die when, from their point of view, life in a distressing or seriously debilitating condition is no longer worthwhile. Different patients will decide differently under relevantly similar circumstances because different patients have different goals and different values. These goals and values ought to be respected. It would be quite inappropriate, in my view, to try to devise uniform and objective criteria as to when a competent patient should or should not undergo a particular life-

[37] John Stuart Mill: 'On Liberty' in E. A. Burtt (ed.): *The English Philosophers from Bacon to Mill* (New York: Modern Library, 1939), 949–1041.
[38] KNMG, 'Policy Statement on Euthanasia'.

sustaining treatment.[39] No objective determination could be adequate because persons have a primary interest in self-determination, that is, in choosing and pursuing their particular plans for life—and death. It is self-determination which is central to what it is to be a moral agent or a person; to deprive a person of control over her own living and dying—in an area where this does not cause harm to others—shows disrespect for that person and is, other things being equal, wrong.

Indeed, it is widely recognized that it is this capacity for self-determination or autonomy which distinguishes normal adult persons not only from most non-human animals, but also from those human beings who never have been, and never will be, autonomous. The latters' interests are necessarily exhausted by their well-being. The formers' are not.

*Infants and patients who have never been competent*   Infants—like some severely retarded or brain-damaged patients—are not competent and cannot make decisions for themselves. They are not 'persons' in Michael Tooley's sense of the term, and cannot have a preference for, or interest in, continued life. Rather, infants are more like foetuses than normal adults. They do not have a 'right to life' and killing them is not directly wrong. This does not mean, though, that it is not normally a good thing to keep handicapped infants and other non-competent patients alive—at least if their lives are likely to be pleasant ones.[40] On the other hand, if the future holds little but suffering and frustrated desires for such a patient, then it would be directly wrong to sustain her life.[41]

*Formerly competent patients*   The other important category is the non-competent patient who, unlike an infant, once was competent or a 'person'. If there are previously expressed wishes, they should—other things being equal—be acted on. This is an extension of Mill's principle, but not a major one. It would ensure that not only the patient's own understanding of well-being is respected, but also her interest in self-determination. We must consider, too, the good effect this will have on the peace of mind of other persons if they can expect

[39] See also President's Commission: *Deciding to Forego Life-sustaining Treatment*, 26–7.
[40] See also R. M. Hare: 'Survival of the Weakest', in S. Gorovitz *et al.* (eds.): *Moral Problems in Medicine* (Englewood Cliffs, NJ: Prentice Hall, 1976), 364–9.
[41] Kuhse and Singer: *Should the Baby Live?* esp. Ch. 7.

that their wishes will be followed in the event of their losing their competence.

If there are no previously expressed wishes, and there is no prospect of the patient recovering competence, the overriding principle should, other things being equal, be the patient's well-being and the prevention of pointless suffering.

## 5.34    Conclusion

Everything I have said so far could be taken to apply both to refraining from preventing death and to killing. Since, as I have argued throughout this book, there is no intrinsic moral difference between killing and letting die, I believe that there will be times when it is better that a patient be killed rather than allowed to die—either because the process of dying involves much unnecessary suffering[42] or because a competent patient asks her doctor for help in dying.

Whilst much more would need to be said to substantiate these points, a quality-of-life ethic based on principles such as the above is ultimately morally defensible. What is *not* morally defensible, though, is the way in which implicit quality-of-life decisions are currently often carried out. If it is, for example, morally defensible to let certain handicapped infants die because infants, like foetuses, do not have a 'right to life', it is not morally defensible to subject them to unnecessary suffering: to withhold so-called 'extraordinary' means of treatment and to then stand by as nature takes her sometimes cruel course. For even if infants do not have a 'right to life', as Tooley's analysis suggests—to the extent that they are capable of experiencing pain and discomfort, they can have a desire not to experience discomfort, not to experience pain. This means that it may not be wrong, other things being equal, to painlessly kill an infant, but wrong to let an infant die under distressing circumstances.

When the Nuer, an East African tribe, saw a need to do away with malformed or otherwise defective infants, they did it by classifying these infants as 'hippopotamuses', mistakenly born to human parents. These infants were put into the river, their natural habitat. This was not terminating the lives of Nuer infants, it was doing what was appropriate for young hippopotamuses; and Nuer morality, prohibiting the taking of tribal life, could emerge unscathed.[43]

---

[42] Kuhse: 'Death by Non-feeding'.

[43] I owe this example to Beauchamp and Childress: *Principles in Biomedical Ethics*, 121.

When we refrain from preventing the deaths of handicapped infants, comatose patients, and the terminally ill and suffering, by classifying the means necessary for keeping them alive as 'extraordinary', 'not medically indicated', 'disproportionately burdensome', and so on, we are resorting to an equally spurious device in order to preserve our sanctity-of-life ethics unscathed. If we want to go beyond definitional ploys, we must accept responsibility for making life and death decisions on the basis of the quality or kind of life in question: we must drop the 'sanctity-of-life' doctrine and work out a quality-of-life ethic instead.

# BIBLIOGRAPHY

Abelard, P., *Peter Abelard's Ethics*. D. E. Luscombe (ed. and trans.). Oxford: Clarendon Press, 1971.

Abrams, N., 'Active and Passive Euthanasia'. *Philosophy* 53 (1978), 257–63.

American Medical Association, 'The Physician and the Dying Patient'. Policy Statement adopted by the House of Delegates on 4 Dec. 1973.

——, 'Withholding or Withdrawing Life Prolonging Medical Treatment'. Policy Statement of the Council on Ethical and Judicial Affairs, 15 Mar. 1986.

Anderson, W. F., 'The Elderly at the End of Life'. In S. Lack and R. Lamerton (eds.): *The Hour of Our Death*, 8–18. London: Chapman, 1974.

Anglican Church Information Office, *On Dying Well: An Anglican Contribution to the Debate on Euthanasia*. Church Information Office, 1979.

Anscombe, G. E. M., *Intention*. Oxford: Basil Blackwell, 1958.

——, 'Modern Moral Philosophy'. *Philosophy*, 33 (1958) 1–19.

——, 'A Note on Mr. Bennett'. *Analysis* 26 (1966), 208.

——, 'Two Kinds of Error in Action'. In J. J. Thomson and G. Dworkin (eds.): *Ethics*, 279–89. New York: Harper & Row, 1968.

——, 'War and Murder'. In R. Wasserstrom (ed.): *War and Morality*, Belmont: Wadsworth Publishing Co., 1970.

Aquinas, T., *Summa Theologiae*, II, ii, question 64, article 5.

——, *Summa Theologiae*, II, ii, question 64, article 7.

D'Arcy, E., *Human Acts*. Oxford: Clarendon Press, 1963.

Aristotle, 'Politics'. In R. McKeon (ed.): *The Basic Works of Aristotle*. New York: Random House, 1941, 1127–316.

Australian Medical Association, Submission to the Law Reform Commission of Western Australia, 8 June 1982.

Barth, K., *Church Dogmatics*, vol. 3. Edinburgh: Clark, 1961.

Beauchamp, T. L. and J. F. Childress, *Principles of Biomedical Ethics*. New York: Oxford University Press, 1979.

Bennett, J., 'Whatever the Consequences'. In J. J. Thomson and G. Dworkin (eds.): *Ethics*, 211–36. New York: Harper & Row, 1968.

——, 'Morality and Consequences'. In S. M. McMurrin (ed.): *The Tanner Lectures on Human Values*, vol. 2, 47–116. Salt Lake City: University of Utah Press and Cambridge University Press, 1981.

Bentham, J., *An Introduction to The Principles of Morals and Legislation*. New York, Hafner Publishing Co., 1948.

Boyle, J. M., Jr., 'On Killing and Letting Die'. *New Scholasticism* 51 (1977), 433–53.

——, 'Toward Understanding the Principle of Double Effect'. *Ethics* 90 (1980), 527–38.

Brandt, R. B., *Ethical Theory*. Englewood Cliffs, NJ: Prentice Hall, 1959.

British Medical Journal., Editorial: 'Withholding Treatment in Infancy'. *British Medical Journal*, 1 (1981), 925–6.

Brody, H., *Ethical Discussions in Medicine*. Boston: Little, Brown, 1976.

Burton, A. W., *Medical Ethics and the Law*. Glebe: Australasian Medical Publishing Co., 1979.

Byrne, P. W. and M. J. Stogre, 'Agathanasia and the Care of the Dying'. In J. Thomas (ed.): *Matters of Life and Death*, 98–104. Toronto: Samuel Stevens, 1978.

Callahan, O., 'The Sanctity of Life'. In D. R. Cutler (ed.): *Updating Life and Death*, 181–223. Boston: Beacon Press, 1969.

Cameron, C. S., *The Truth about Cancer*. Englewood Cliffs, NJ: Prentice Hall, 1956.

Casey, J., 'Actions and Consequences'. In John Casey (ed.): *Morality and Moral Reasoning*, 155–205. London: Methuen, 1971.

Catholic University of America., *New Catholic Encyclopaedia*, vol. 4. New York: McGraw-Hill, 1976.

Chisholm, R. M., 'The Structure of Intention'. *The Journal of Philosophy* 67 (1970), 633–47.

Colen, B. D., *Karen Ann Quinlan: Living and Dying in the Age of Eternal Life*. Los Angeles: Nash, 1976.

Collins, V. J., 'Limits of Medical Responsibility in Prolonging Life'. *Journal of the American Medical Association* 206 (1968), 389–92.

Crane, D., *The Sanctity of Social Life: Physicians' Treatment of Critically Ill Patients*. New York: Russell Sage Foundation, 1975.

Danner Clouser, K., 'The "Sanctity of Life": An Analysis of a Concept'. *Annals of Internal Medicine* 78 (1973), 110–125.

Davidson, D., 'Actions, Reasons and Causes'. *The Journal of Philosophy* 60 (1963), 685–700.

——, 'The Logical Form of Action Sentences'. In Nicholas Rescher (ed.): *The Logic of Decision and Action*, 81–120. Pittsburgh: University of Pittsburgh Press, 1967.

——, 'Causal Relations'. In Myles Brand (ed.): *The Nature of Causation*, 353–67. Chicago, University of Illinois Press, 1976.

Davis, N., 'The Priority of Avoiding Harm'. In B. Steinbock (ed.): *Killing and Letting Die*, 173–215. Englewood Cliffs, NJ: Prentice Hall, 1980.

Department of Health and Social Security, *Care of the Child with Spina Bifida*. London: HMSO, 1973.

Devine, P. E., *The Ethics of Homicide*. Ithaca: Cornell University Press, 1978.

Dinello, D., 'On Killing and Letting Die'. In Bonnie Steinbock (ed.): *Killing and Letting Die*, 128–31. Englewood Cliffs, NJ: Prentice Hall, 1980.

Donagan, A. *The Theory of Morality*. Chicago and London: The University of Chigago Press, 1977.

Duff, R. A., 'Intentionally Killing the Innocent'. *Analysis* 34 (1973), 16–19.

——, 'Absolute Principles and Double Effect'. *Analysis* 36 (1976), 68–80.

——, 'Intention, Responsibility, and Double Effect'. *The Philosophical Quarterly* 32 (1982), 1–16.

Duff, R. S. and A. G. M. Campbell, 'Moral and Ethical Dilemmas: Seven Years into the Debate about Human Ambiguity'. *Annals of the American Academy of Political and Social Science* 447 (1980), 19–28.

——, 'Moral and Ethical Dilemmas in the Special-care Nursery'. *New England Journal of Medicine* 289 (1973), 890–4.

Eckstein, Hatcher and Slater, Medical Practice—'New Horizons in Medical Ethics: Severely Malformed Children—a Taperecorded Discussion'. *British Medical Journal*, 2 (1973), 294–9.

Farley, M., 'A Response to Dr. Duff'. *Reflection* 72 (1975), 11–12.

Festinger, L., *A Theory of Cognitive Dissonance*: Stanford: Stanford University Press, 1957.

Finnis, J., 'The Rights and Wrongs of Abortion: A Reply to Judith Thomson'. *Philosophy and Public Affairs* 2 (1973), 117–45.

Fitzgerald, P. J., 'Acting and Refraining'. *Analysis* 27 (1973), 133–9.

Fletcher, G. P., 'Prolonging Life: Some Legal Considerations'. In Bonnie Steinbock (ed.): *Killing and Letting Die*, 45–55. Englewood Cliffs, NJ: Prentice Hall, 1980.

Fletcher, J., *Morals and Medicine*. Boston: Beacon Press, 1954.

——, 'Indicators of Humanhood: A Tentative Profile of Man'. *Hastings Center Report* 2 (1972), 1–4.

——, *Humanhood: Essays in Biomedical Ethics*. Buffalo, N.Y.: Prometheus Books, 1980.

Foot, P., 'Moral Arguments'. *Mind* 67 (1958), 502–13.

——, 'The Problem of Abortion and the Doctrine of Double Effect'. In Bonnie Steinbock (ed.): *Killing and Letting Die*, 156–65. Englewood Cliffs, NJ: Prentice Hall, 1980.

Fost, N., 'Putting Hospitals on Notice'. *Hastings Center Report* 12 (1982), 5–8.

Frankena, W. K., 'The Ethics of Respect for Life'. In S. F. Barker (ed.): *Respect for Life in Medicine, Philosophy, and the Law*, 24–62. Baltimore: Johns Hopkins University Press, 1977.

——, 'McCormick and the Traditional Distinction'. In R. McCormick and P. Ramsey (eds.): *Doing Evil to Achieve Good*, 145–64. Chicago: Loyola University Press, 1978.

Freeman, J., 'Is there a Right to Die—Quickly?'. *Journal of Pediatrics* 80 (1972), 904–5.

——, 'The Short-sighted Treatment of Myelomeningocele: A Long-term Case Report'. *Pediatrics* 53:3 (1974), 311–13.

Frey, R. G., 'Some Aspects of the Doctrine of Double Effect'. *Canadian Journal of Philosophy* 5 (1975), 259–83.

Fried, C., *Right and Wrong*. Cambridge, Mass.: Harvard University Press, 1978.

Geddes, L., 'On the Intrinsic Wrongness of Killing Innocent People'. *Analysis* 33 (1973), 93–7.

Glover, J., *Causing Death and Saving Lives*. Harmondsworth: Penguin, 1977.

Goldman, A. I., *A Theory of Human Action*. Englewood Cliffs, NJ: Prentice Hall, 1970.

Goldman, H., 'Killing, Letting Die and Euthanasia'. *Analysis* 40 (1980), 224.

Gorovitz, S. *et al* (eds.). Editorial comment: 'Spina Bifida'. In *Moral Problems in Medicine*, 341–2. Englewood Cliffs, NJ: Prentice Hall, 1976.

Gould, J. and Lord Craigmyle (eds.), *Your Death Warrant?* London: Chapman, 1971.

Graham, G., 'Doing Something Intentionally and Moral Responsibility'. *Canadian Journal of Philosophy* 11 (1981), 667–77.

Green, O. H., 'Killing and Letting Die'. *American Philosophical Quarterly* 17 (1980), 195–204.

Grisez, G., *Abortion: the Myths, the Realities, and the Arguments*. New York: Corpus Books, 1970.

——, 'Toward a Consistent Natural Law Ethics of Killing'. *American Journal of Jurisprudence* 15 (1970), 64–96.

Gruzalski, B., 'Killing and Letting Die'. *Mind* 40 (1981), 91–8.

Gustafson, J. M., 'Mongolism, Parental Desires, and the Right to Life'. In Robert F. Weir (ed.): *Ethical Issues in Death and Dying*, 145–72. New York: Columbia University Press, 1977.

Habermas, J., *Legitimation Crisis*, T. McCarthy (trans.). Boston: Beacon Press, 1975.

Häring, B., *Medical Ethics*. Notre Dame, Ind.: Fides Publ., 1973.

Hanink, J. G., 'Some Light on Double Effect'. *Analysis* 35 (1975), 147–51.

Hare, R. M., *The Language of Morals*. London: Oxford University Press, 1952.

——, *Freedom and Reason*. Oxford: Oxford University Press, 1963.

——,'Euthanasia: A Christian View'. *Philosophic Exchange* II (1975), 43–52.

——, 'Survival of the Weakest'. In S. Gorovitz *et al*. (eds.): *Moral Problems in Medicine*, 364–9. Englewood Cliffs, NJ: Prentice Hall, 1976.

——, *Moral Thinking*. Oxford: Clarendon Press, 1981.

Harris, J., *Violence and Responsibility*. London: Routledge and Kegan Paul, 1980.

——, 'Bad Samaritans Cause Harm'. *The Philosophical Quarterly* 32 (1982), 60–9.

——, *The Value of Life*. London: Routledge and Kegan Paul, 1985.

Harkness, G., *The Sources of Western Morality*. New York: Charles Scribner's Sons, 1954.

Hart, H. L. A., *Punishment and Responsibility*. Oxford: Clarendon Press, 1968.

Hart, H. L. A. and A. M. Honoré, *Causation in the Law*. London: Oxford University Press, 1959.

Hastings Center, Editorial Comment: 'Doctors "Not Guilty" of Prolonging Life at Any Cost'. *Hastings Center Report* 9 (1979), 2–3.

Heenan, Cardinal J., 'A Fascinating Story'. In S. Lack and R. Lamerton (eds.): *The Hour of Our Death: A Record of the Conference on the Care of the Dying held in London, 1973*, 1–7. London: Chapman, 1974.

Hughes, G. J., 'Killing and Letting Die'. *The Month* 2nd n.s. (1975), 42–5.

——, 'Commentary "Helga Kuhse: Extraordinary Means and the Sanctity of Life" '. *Journal of Medical Ethics* 7 (1981), 79–81.

Hume, D., *An Enquiry Concerning Human Understanding*. New York: Collier Books, 1962.

Jackson, F., 'Review of Myles Brand (ed.): *The Nature of Causation*'. Journal of Symbolic Logic 42 (1982), 470–3.

Jonsen, A. R. and G. Lister, 'Life Support Systems'. In Warren T. Reich (ed.): *Encyclopedia of Bioethics*, vol. 2, 841–8. New York: Free Press, 1978.

Kadish, S. H., 'Respect for Life and Regard for Rights in the Criminal Law'. In S. F. Barker (ed.): *Respect for Life in Medicine, Philosophy, and the Law*, 63–101. Baltimore: Johns Hopkins University Press, 1977.

Karnofsky, D. A., 'Why Prolong the Life of a Patient with Advanced Cancer?'. *Cancer Journal for Clinicians* 10 (1960), 9–11.

Keane, H., *A Primer of Moral Philosophy*. Catholic Social Guild, Oxford. New York: P. J. Kenny & Sons, n.d.

Kelly, G., *Medico-moral Problems*. St Louis: The Catholic Hospital Association of the United States and Canada, 1958.

Keyserlingk, E. W., *Sanctity of Life or Quality of Life* (in the context of ethics, medicine, and law). Study written for the Law Reform Commission of Canada. Ottawa: Law Reform Commission, 1979.

KNMG (Royal Dutch Association of Medicine), 'Policy Statement on Euthanasia'. *Medisch Contact* 39 : 31 (3 August 1985).

Kohl, M., 'The Sanctity-of-Life Principle'. In Marvin Kohl (ed.): *The Morality of Killing: Sanctity-of-Life, Abortion and Euthanasia*, 3–23. London: Peter Owen, 1974.

Kuhse, H, 'Extraordinary Means and the Intentional Termination of Life'. *Social Science and Medicine* 15F (1981), 117–21.

——, 'Extraordinary Means and the Sanctity of Life'. *Journal of Medical Ethics* 7 (1981), 74–82.

——, 'An Ethical Approach to IVF and ET: What Ethics is All About'. In W.

Walters and P. Singer (eds): *Test-tube Babies*, 22–35. Melbourne: Oxford University Press, 1982.

——, 'A Modern Myth: That Letting Die is not the Intentional Causation of Death: Some Reflections on the Trial and Acquittal of Dr Leonard Arthur'. *Journal of Applied Philosophy* 1:1 (1984), 21–38.

——, 'Interests'. *Journal of Medical Ethics*, 11 (1985), 146–9.

——, 'Death by Non-feeding: Not in the Baby's Best Interests', *Journal of Medical Humanities and Bioethics* 7:3 (1986).

—— and P. Singer, *Should the Baby Live? The Problem of Handicapped Infants*. Oxford: Oxford University Press, 1985.

Lack S. and R. Lamerton (eds.), *The Hour of Our Death*, A record of the conference on the care of the dying held in London, 1973. London: Chapman, 1974.

Ladd, J., 'Positive and Negative Euthanasia'. In M. D. Bayles and D. M. High (eds.): *Medical Treatment of the Dying: Moral Issues*, 105–27. Cambridge, Mass.: Hall & Co., 1978.

Lecky, W. E. H., *History of European Morals from Augustus to Charlemagne*, vol. ii, 11th edn. London: Longmans Green & Co., 1894.

Linacre Centre Working Party, *Euthanasia and Clinical Practice: Trends, Principles and Alternatives*. London: The Linacre Centre, 1982.

Locke, D. 'Absolutism and Consequentialism: No Contest'. *Analysis* 41 (1981), 101–6.

Locke, J., 'An Essay Concerning the True Original, Extent and End of Civil Government'. In E. Barker (ed.) *Social Contract*, 1–144. London: Oxford University Press, 1971.

Lorber, J., 'Early Results of Selective Treatment for Spina Bifida Cystica'. *British Medical Journal* 4 (1973), 201–4.

——, 'Ethical Problems in the Management of Myelomeningocele and Hydrocephalus'. *Journal of the Royal College of Physicians* 10 (1975), 47–60.

——, ' "Commentary I and reply" to John Harris: "Ethical Problems in the Management of Some Severely Handicapped Children" '. *Journal of Medical Ethics* 7, (1981), pp. 120–2.

Lyon, J., *Playing God in the Nursery*. New York: Norton, 1985.

McAllister, J. B., *Ethics with Special Application to the Medical and Nursing Professions*, 2nd. edn. Philadelphia: 1955.

McCloskey, H. J., 'The Right to Life', *Mind* 84 (1975), 403–25.

McCormick, R. A., 'To Save or Let Die: The Dilemma of Modern Medicine', *The Journal of the American Medical Association* 229 (1974), 172–6.

——, 'The Quality of Life, The Sanctity of Life'. *Hastings Center Report* 8 (1978), 30–6.

MacIntyre, A., 'Why is the Search for the Foundation of Ethics so Frustrating?'. *Hastings Center Report* 9 (1979), 16–22.

Mackie, J. L., *The Cement of the Universe*. London: Oxford University Press, 1974.

——, 'Causes and Conditions'. In Ernest Sosa (ed.): *Causation and Conditionals*, 15–38. London: Oxford University Press, 1975.

——, *Ethics: Inventing Right and Wrong*. Harmondsworth: Penguin, 1977.

Mangan, J., 'An Historical Analysis of the Principle of Double Effect'. *Theological Studies* 10 (1949), 41–61.

May, W., 'Ethics and Human Identity: The Challenge of the New Biology'. *Horizons* 3 (1976), 35–7.

Meiland, J. W., *The Nature of Intention*. London: Methuen, 1970.

Mill, J. S., *A System of Logic*. London: Longman's, 1959.

——, 'On Liberty'. In E. A. Burtt (ed.): *The English Philosophers from Bacon to Mill*, 949–1041. New York: Modern Library, 1939.

——, *Utilitarianism*. London: Collins, 1968.

Moore, G. E., *Principia Ethica*. Cambridge: Cambridge University Press, 1978.

More, T., *Utopia*. Cambridge: Cambridge University Press, 1908.

Morillo, C. R., 'Doing, Refraining, and the Strenuousness of Morality'. *American Philosophical Quarterly* 14 (1977), 29–39.

Morison, R. S., 'Death: Process or Event?'. *Science* 173 (1971), 694–8.

Nagel, T., 'Death'. In James Rachels (ed.): *Moral Problems*, 2nd. edn., 401–9. New York: Harper & Row, 1975.

——, 'The Limits of Objectivity'. In S. McMurrin (ed.): *The Tanner Lectures on Human Values*, vol. i, pp. 76–139. Cambridge: Cambridge University Press, 1980.

——, 'War and Massacre'. *Philosophy and Public Affairs* 1(1972), 123–44.

Nicholson, R., 'Should the Patient be Allowed to Die?'. *Journal of Medical Ethics* (1975), 5–9.

Pius XII, *Acta Apostolicae Sedis* 43 (1951).

——, *Acta Apostolicae Sedis* (1957).

Plato, *The Republic*, trans. H. D. P. Lee. Harmondsworth: Penguin, 1972.

President's Commission for the Study of Ethical Problems in Medicine and Biomedical and Behavioral Research, *Deciding to Forego Life-sustaining Treatment, Ethical Medical & Legal Issues in Treatment Decisions*, Washington, D.C.: GPO.

Primatt, H., *A Dissertation on the Duty of Mercy and the Sin of Cruelty to Brute Animals*. London, 1776.

Rabkin, M. T. *et al.*, 'Orders Not to Resuscitate'. *The New England Journal of Medicine* 295 (1976), 364–6.

Rachels, J., 'Euthanasia, Killing and Letting Die'. In John Ladd (ed.): *Ethical Issues Relating to Life and Death*, 146–63. New York: Oxford University Press, 1979.

——, 'Killing and Starving to Death'. *Philosophy* 54 (1979), 159–71.

——, 'Active and Passive Euthanasia'. In Bonnie Steinbock (ed.): *Killing and Letting Die*, 63–8. Englewood Cliffs, NJ: Prentice Hall, 1980.

——, 'Euthanasia'. In Tom Regan (ed.): *Matters of Life and Death*, 28–66. New York: Random House, 1980.

——, *The End of Life*. Oxford: Oxford University Press, 1986.

Ramsey, P., 'The Morality of Abortion'. In D. L. Labby (ed.): *Life or Death*, 60–93. Seattle: University of Washington Press, 1968.

——, *The Patient as Person*. New Haven: Yale University Press, 1970.

——, 'Prolonged Dying: Not Medically Indicated', *Hastings Center Report* 6 (1976), 14–17.

——, 'Euthanasia and Dying Well Enough'. *Linacre Quarterly* 4 (1977), 60–93.

——, *Ethics at the Edges of Life*. New Haven: Yale University Press, 1978.

Robertson, J. A., 'Dilemma in Danville'. *The Hastings Center Report* 11 (1981), 5–8.

Rosenbaum, E. H., *Living with Cancer*. New York: Praeger, 1975.

Rostand, J., *Humanly Possible: A Biologist's Notes on the Future of Mankind*. New York: Saturday Review Press, 1973.

Russell, B., 'On the Relative Strictness of Negative and Positive Duties'. In B. Steinbock (ed.): *Killing and Letting Die*, 215–31. Englewood Cliffs NJ: Prentice Hall, 1980.

Sacred Congregation for the Doctrine of the Faith, *Declaration on Euthanasia*. Vatican City, 1980.

Schopenhauer, A., *The World as Will and Representation*, trans. E. J. F. Payne. New York: 1969.

Schweitzer, A., *Civilization and Ethics*, 3rd. edn. London: Black, 1949.

Seneca, 'De Ira'. In T. E. Page *et al.* (eds): *Seneca Moral Essays*, trans. J. W. Basore. vol. i. London: Heinemann, 1958.

——, '58th Letter to Lucilius'. In T. E. Page *et al.* (eds.): *Seneca: Ad Lucilium Epistulae Morales*, trans. R. M. Gummere, vol. i. London: Heinemann, 1961.

Shaffer, J. *Philosophy of Mind*. Englewood Cliffs, NJ: Prentice Hall, 1968.

Shaw, A., T. G. Randolph, and B. Menard, 'Ethical Issues in Pediatric Surgery: A National Survey of Pediatricians and Pediatric Surgeons' *Pediatrics* 60 (1977), 588–99.

Shaw, A., 'Dilemmas of Informed Consent in Children'. *New England Journal of Medicine* 289 (1973), 885–90.

——, 'Doctor, Do We Have a Choice?'. *New York Times Magazine*, 1972, p. 54.

Sidgwick, H., *The Ethics of T. H. Green, H. Spencer, and J. Martineau*, London: Macmillan, 1902.

——, *The Methods of Ethics*, 7th edn. London: Macmillan, 1907.

Sikora, R. I., 'Killing and Letting Die: Twelve Cases', unpublished paper.

Singer, P., *Practical Ethics*. Cambridge: Cambridge University Press, 1979.
——, *The Expanding Circle*. New York: Farrar, Straus & Giroux, 1981.
——, H. Kuhse, and C. Singer, 'The Treatment of Newborn Infants with Major Handicaps: A Survey of Obstetricians and Paediatricians in Victoria'. *The Medical Journal of Australia* 2:6 (1983), 274–9.
Smart, J. J. C., 'An Outline of a System of Utilitarian Ethics'. In J. J. C. Smart and B. Williams: *Utilitarianism For and Against*, 3–67. Cambridge: Cambridge University Press, 1973.
Steinbock, B., 'The Intentional Termination of Life'. In B. Steinbock (ed.): *Killing and Letting Die*, 69–77. Englewood Cliffs, NJ: Prentice Hall, 1980.
——, (ed.), *Killing and Letting Die*. Englewood Cliffs, NJ Prentice Hall, 1980.
Strand, J. G., 'The "Living Will": The Right to Death with Dignity'. *Western Reserve Law Review* 26 (1976), 485–526.
Sumner, L. W., *Abortion and Moral Theory*. Princeton: Princeton University Press, 1981.
Swinyard, C. A., *Decision Making and the Defective Newborn*: Proceedings of a Conference on Spina Bifida and Ethics. Springfield: Charles C. Thomas, 1978.
Temkin, O., 'Respect for Life in the History of Medicine'. In S. F. Barker (ed.): *Respect for Life in Medicine, Philosophy and the Law*, 1–23. Baltimore: Johns Hopkins University Press, 1977.
—— and C. L. Temkin (eds.), *Ancient Medicine: Selected Papers of Ludwig Edelstein*. Baltimore: Johns Hopkins University Press, 1967.
Thomson, J. J., 'The Time of a Killing'. *Journal of Philosophy* 68 (1971), 115–32.
——, 'Rights and Death'. In Marshall Cohen *et al.* (eds.): *The Rights and Wrongs of Abortion*, 146–59. Princeton: University Press, 1974.
——, *Acts and Other Events*. Ithaca: Cornell University Press, 1977.
Tooley, M., 'An Irrelevant Consideration: Killing versus Letting Die'. In Bonnie Steinbock (ed.): *Killing and Letting Die*, 56–62. Englewood Cliffs, NJ: Prentice Hall, 1980.
——, *Abortion and Infanticide*. Oxford: Clarendon Press, 1983.
Trammel, R. L., 'Saving Life and Taking Life'. *The Journal of Philosophy* 72 (1975), 131–7.
——, 'The Presumption against Taking Life'. *The Journal of Medicine and Philosophy* 3 (1978), 53–67.
Uniacke, S., 'The Doctrine of Double Effect'. *The Thomist* 48:2 (1984) 188–218.
US Government, Child Abuse and Neglect Prevention and Treatment Program 45CIR; Proposed Rule, *Federal Register*, vol. 49, no. 238.
US Government, Department of Health and Human Services, Office for Civil Rights: 'Notice to Health Care Providers'. 18 May 1982; reprinted in *Hastings Center Report* 12, (1982), 6.

US Supreme Court of New Jersey, *70 N.J. In the Matter of Karen Quinlan, An Alleged Incompetent*, Argued 26 January 1976, decided 31 March 1976. Reprinted in B. Steinbock (ed.): *Killing and Letting Die*, 23–44. Englewood Cliffs, NJ: Prentice Hall, 1980.

Veatch, R. M., 'The Whole-brain-oriented Concept of Death: An Outmoded Philosophical Formulation'. *Journal of Thanatology* 3 (1975), 13–30.

——, *Death, Dying and the Biological Revolution*. New Haven: Yale University Press, 1976.

——, *Case Studies in Medical Ethics*. Cambridge, Mass.: Harvard University Press, 1979.

Walters, W. and P. Singer, *Test-tube Babies*. Melbourne: Oxford University Press, 1982.

Walton, D. N., *On Defining Death*. Montreal: McGill–Queen's University Press, 1979.

Warren, M. A., 'On the Moral and Legal Status of Abortion'. *The Monist* 57 (1973), 43–62.

Weber, L., *Who Shall Live?* New York: Paulist Press, 1976.

Weinryb, E., 'Omission and Responsibility'. *The Philosophical Quarterly* 30 (1980), 1–18.

Williams, B., 'The Makropulos Case: Reflections on the Tedium of Immortality'. In James Rachels (ed.): *Moral Problems*, 2nd edn., 410–28. New York: Harper & Row, 1975.

Williams, G., *The Sanctity of Life and the Criminal Law*. London: Faber & Faber, 1958.

Wilson, J. B., *Death by Decision*. Philadelphia: Westminster Press, 1975.

Woodward, K. L., 'The Ethics of Miracles'. *Newsweek*, 19 September 1977, p. 57.

World Medical Assembly, 'Statement on Terminal Illness and Boxing: 35th Medical Assembly, Venice (Italy) October 1983. *Medical Journal of Australia*, 140 (1984), 431.

World Medical Association, Declaration of Geneva. (Medical vow adopted by the General Assembly in September 1948. Amended by the 22nd World Medical Assembly, Sydney, Australia, 1968.)

Zachary, R. B., 'Ethical and Social Aspects of Spina Bifida'. *Lancet* 2 (1968), 274–76.

——, 'The Neonatal Surgeon'. *British Medical Journal* 4 (1976) 866–69.

# INDEX